Siobhan Miller, the parent of three boys, is an experienced hypnobirthing teacher and founder of The Positive Birth Company, which aims to empower expectant parents and birth partners with knowledge and equip them with the tools they need to create positive birth experiences.

HYPNOBIRTHING

PRACTICAL WAYS TO MAKE YOUR BIRTH BETTER

Siobhan Miller

Founder of The Positive Birth Company

PIATKUS

PIATKUS

First published in Great Britain in 2019 by Piatkus
This reissue edition published in Great Britain in 2023 by Piatkus

5 7 9 10 8 6 4

A CIP catalogue record for this book
is available from the British Library.

ISBN 978-0-349-43517-6

Illustrations on pages 3 and 43 © Louise Turpin
Illustrations on page 7 © Josephine Dellow

Typeset in Calluna by M Rules
Printed and bound by Clays Ltd, Elcograf S.p.A.

Papers used by Piatkus are from well-managed forests
and other responsible sources.

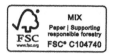

Piatkus
An imprint of
Little, Brown Book Group
Carmelite House
50 Victoria Embankment
London EC4Y 0DZ

An Hachette UK Company
www.hachette.co.uk

www.littlebrown.co.uk

For Oisin, Arlo, Ailbe and the
little person not yet born.
Thank you for choosing me.
Being your mama is the greatest
honour of my life.

Contents

About Me

Hello! I'm Siobhan and besides being the author of this book, I'm also a hypnobirthing teacher, the founder of The Positive Birth Company and, best of all, a mum to my three wild boys. I'm on a mission to make hypnobirthing more accessible, and I hope this book will enable me to reach more people around the world, helping them to have better births.

Before we begin, I thought I'd share a little of my personal experience with birth and how I came to be such a huge advocate for hypnobirthing.

My first son was born when I was just twenty-one, and, although I attended the free antenatal classes at my local hospital, I was not very informed when it came to many aspects of birth. I wanted a vaginal birth and learnt some effective breathing techniques, but when I was offered an induction at forty weeks and eight days I naively thought that meant I would get to meet my baby sooner, effectively speeding up the waiting game without any negative consequences. I knew very little about the risks associated with induction and had no idea I could decline.

Instead of the quick, straightforward birth I had dreamt of, my induction took two days and involved almost every form of pain relief and intervention that had been mentioned in our antenatal classes. During my induction I spent all my time in a brightly lit hospital room with a TV on in the corner, which at some point was playing a show about plastic surgery gone wrong! I was advised not to eat in case I ended up needing a caesarean. After two days without food or sleep, it's little wonder I needed assistance. I was taken to theatre in the early hours for an unplanned caesarean as my baby was showing signs of distress and I was exhausted, but once I was in theatre (having had my epidural topped up so I could feel nothing) the consultant used forceps to turn my baby's head and I was given the opportunity to push him out. Which I did. It was an overwhelming moment of relief when he was placed on my chest. I remember him raising his little head and looking me square in the eyes. I remember thinking 'I'm sure babies aren't meant to be able to hold their heads up!' It was a moment I will never forget. I wasn't traumatised by the experience, but it was certainly a frightening one and not a birth I'd describe as particularly positive or empowering. In the months that followed my first son's birth I suffered with severe anxiety and was full of fear about his well-being, which now, on reflection, I attribute to the birth experience. At the time I knew very little about what birth was like, other than what I'd seen on the TV – and using that as a benchmark my experience, sadly, seemed pretty average.

Fast forward seven years and this is where it gets good! I was pregnant with my second baby and had seen and read enough to know that birth could be different: a positive, magical experience and something to be cherished. So, I signed up to a hypnobirthing course and, without exaggeration, it changed my life. Not only did I feel excited about my upcoming birth but, importantly, I was able to properly process and put to rest what had happened in my previous birth. With my new-found knowledge I was able to understand why so many things had panned out the way they had, and, as a result, felt confident that the same thing would not happen again. I was able to let go of all my fears.

My partner, who initially had been very sceptical about attending a hypnobirthing class, was on board after the first session and an advocate after the second; it was all so logical and scientific. It made absolute sense. In fact, I'd go as far as saying that it's pretty much impossible *not* to get on board with it. You don't need to subscribe to any particular school of thought or be a particular kind of person; hypnobirthing is for every person who is preparing to bring a baby into the world, no matter how they plan on doing that. It's as simple as that.

After the course, I planned a home birth – quite the opposite end of the spectrum compared to my theatre birth – and practised all my relaxation techniques. I remember thinking that even if the birth didn't go as I'd hoped, I would still have benefited enormously from the course because I felt so calm, positive and happy in my pregnancy as a result. It was a wonderful time.

I went into labour spontaneously at thirty-nine weeks and six days. My labour was two hours and twenty minutes, start to finish. It was quick and it was intense, but the moment I gave birth on that sofa under the twinkling lights of the Christmas tree I felt the best I had ever felt in my whole life. It was the highest of highs, complete euphoria – I felt invincible! And I rode that high for many weeks afterwards. It really was life-changing – not just the birth experience itself but also the profound impact my positive experience had on the postnatal period that followed. I felt confident and capable, happy and relaxed, and in the best place to enjoy my beautiful baby.

Inspired by this incredible experience, and after completing an MSc in Psychology, I then trained to become a hypnobirthing teacher in 2015 with Katherine Graves and began teaching classes.

In 2016 I had my third baby. This time it was a calm, uncomplicated water birth at my local birth centre. It was such a beautiful and peaceful experience. I describe it as almost uneventful, because there was no drama whatsoever (but of course birthing an actual human is pretty bloody eventful in itself!). If my first birth experience had unfolded like a checklist of all the things that could go 'wrong', my third birth was textbook and followed perfectly the checklist of everything that I had wanted to happen. My second birth was not just a fluke: my third baby confirmed to me the huge positive difference hypnobirthing makes.

I now run hypnobirthing group classes across the UK and remain committed to empowering expectant parents and their birth partners to create positive birth experiences, because birth really does matter and a positive experience offers lifelong benefits for parents, babies and entire families.

In 2017 I made it my mission to make hypnobirthing more affordable, accessible and inclusive, because I strongly believe everyone deserves the best birth possible, as well as the tools to make this a reality. Initially I released a series of free videos on YouTube, then launched the Hypnobirthing Digital Pack – the world's most affordable and accessible online hypnobirthing programme, which is now being used by hundreds of thousands of people around the globe. It was an absolute dream come true to be given the opportunity to write this book and share everything I've learnt in a new format. I knew I didn't want to simply write another book about what hypnobirthing was, so I set out to create an informative and comprehensive handbook that would be enjoyable to read and would equip people with a practical, easy-to-use toolkit that they could use in birth; a book that would actually make their birth better.

My dream is to change the negative narrative around birth, in the hope that this will change the way we approach and think about birth. I want people to go into birth feeling relaxed and positive and come out feeling empowered and strong, confident and capable as they embark on their journey into parenthood. I wrote this book for every type of person and every type of birth. I hope you will read it, enjoy it and then, once finished, pass on its message. By spreading the word, sharing your positive birth story, you're helping to change the world – one birth at a time.

Introduction
What is hypnobirthing and how is it going to help you?

It is likely that you have picked up this book because you're pregnant – or perhaps your partner is – and you've heard the term 'hypnobirthing' thrown around quite a bit, but are not completely sure what it involves or whether it's something you should invest your precious time or money in.

So, firstly, and before we go any further, let me assure you that hypnobirthing does *not* involve being hypnotised and has nothing to do with hippies – or, indeed, hippos! In fact, there is nothing unusual about hypnobirthing at all, besides perhaps the name ... which is ironic. Most modern hypnobirthing teachers will agree that hypnobirthing could really do with a rebrand. There's no doubt the word 'hypno' deters people and leaves them with misconceptions about what hypnobirthing actually is.

I think hypnobirthing can best be described as the psychology of birth. In fact, it's a lot like sports psychology. Just as athletes need to prepare mentally, as well as physically, to improve their performance, there is a similar need for people to prepare psychologically for labour and impending parenthood in order to get the best out of the experience.

Essentially hypnobirthing is a form of antenatal education, an approach to birth that is both evidence-based and logical. You may be surprised to know that it's more scientific than anything else! In this book you will learn about the physiology of birth, and by that I mean how your body works on a muscular and hormonal level when in labour. This should boost your confidence and make it easier to trust that your body really does know what to do. Importantly, you learn how to work *with* your body (rather than unintentionally against it) to ensure the *right* hormones are produced, making labour more efficient and comfortable for you and your baby.

You will discover that being calm and relaxed is key, and that this has a direct and positive impact on how your birth pans out. You will learn how to quickly and easily access a state of deep relaxation using the hypnobirthing toolkit: a combination of breathing techniques, visualisations, guided relaxation exercises, light-touch massage, positive affirmations and various other techniques. You will also learn how to make informed choices using a simple framework, so that you are in a position to navigate your birth – and any twists and turns – with confidence, armed with practical aids that ensure you feel calm and in control throughout.

Crucially, hypnobirthing is not for only one type of birth, just as it's not for only one type of person. Hypnobirthing is for *everyone* with a baby inside their uterus (you don't need to subscribe to any particular school of thought) and for *every* type of birth (from a water birth without intervention or pain relief, through to an unplanned caesarean). Many people come to hypnobirthing wanting a vaginal birth, but I always say that actually the mechanics of *how* a baby enters the world matter little long-term in comparison to how the person *felt* during the experience, because it's the feelings that last a lifetime. This is why a positive birth experience is so important and offers lifelong benefits for parents, babies and entire families. It is well known that a positive birth significantly reduces your risk of experiencing postnatal depression (PND) and post-traumatic stress disorder (PTSD). Giving birth and becoming a parent to a small person is a monumental moment in a person's life, whether it's their first time or fourth time, which is why birth really does matter. As much as parenthood is about winging it, putting some time into preparing for a positive birth is always worth it. In this book you will learn about inductions and caesareans and how you can make *all* births positive using hypnobirthing techniques.

So, what constitutes a positive birth? I believe that a positive birth is a birth experience that leaves you feeling empowered rather than traumatised, a birth in which your wishes are respected, you're listened to, and where you feel calm, confident and informed throughout. Water birth, home birth, induction, caesarean – it's not one particular *type* of birth. All births have the potential to be positive.

The hypnobirthing programme I teach is all about helping expectant parents – and their birth partners – to create these positive birth experiences. It's beneficial for birth partners to learn about hypnobirthing too, as it equips them with practical tools they can use to aid relaxation, a framework to help them ask the right questions, knowledge about how to make the environment conducive for birth and a comprehensive to-do list, so that they know how to best support someone in labour. Hypnobirthing helps birth partners to feel confident, empowered and prepared for the job, rather than feeling nervous and like a spare part in the room. In hypnobirthing we believe giving birth is a team effort and not a one-person job, so make sure you share this book with your birth partner.

Finally, hypnobirthing benefits your baby by ensuring that they have a gentle entry into the world and are met by a parent who feels relaxed, confident and happy. A positive birth gives everyone the best start.

In this book I will cover everything that you would learn on a hypnobirthing course, from start to finish. As you progress through the book and learn more and more, you will feel as though you are completing a course – a fun one, though! This is no boring textbook. I will guide you through the hypnobirthing course I teach, in the order I teach it, chapter by chapter. After reading it, I hope you feel informed, prepared and armed with *everything* you need to create your own amazing birth experience. This book promises to make your birth better!

Becoming a parent is a huge undertaking and it can take its toll both physically and mentally. Growing a human is no mean feat and places significant demands on a person's body. There is also the emotional and psychological impact of assuming this new role, especially as it carries with it such immense and often overwhelming levels of responsibility. It's very common, if not universal, to occasionally mourn one's pre-child life. Then there are the 24/7 demands that need to be met by the new boss who will quite literally throw their toys out of the pram if you fail to deliver what they want in a timely fashion. Throw a shedload of hormones into this messy cocktail and it's not difficult to understand that the transition to parenthood can be tricky. And all this on a few hours of broken sleep.

Sleep deprivation is the shared torture of new parents. Therefore, preparing for this life-changing event is so important. I'll say this more than once: the benefits of hypnobirthing and a positive birth experience extend well beyond the birth itself. What you are going to learn are life skills: tools and techniques you can use to navigate pregnancy, birth and parenthood in the best way possible.

As you read this book, you'll discover that the hypnobirthing programme is really logical – common sense, even. Lots of what

I will talk about is based on scientific understanding of our anatomy, the autonomic nervous system (which controls functions not consciously directed) and the latest evidence-based recommendations for best practice in birth. For those of you who, like me, love a stat or fancy a bit of fact checking, at the back of this book you will find a list of the sources that I reference and recommended further reading.

As you read you will start to realise how so much of what you *think* you know about birth is actually the result of social conditioning. You may well start to feel cheated, even lied to. I get it – I've felt that too. You might feel angry and frustrated and even sad for the hundreds of people who give birth every day *without* this knowledge; who aren't properly informed and ultimately miss out on having what can be the most incredible experience of their life. You'll say to yourself – and to anyone else who will listen – 'But *everyone* should know this stuff!' This is *exactly* how I feel too, and precisely why this book has come to be in your hands today.

It's worth mentioning that hypnobirthing isn't a 'new' thing. If anything, it is a rejection of the 'new' over-medicalised approach to birth and a *return* to how birth used to be. Medical and technological advances, coupled with the introduction of the NHS, have meant that more and more people have gone to hospital to give birth over the years, until it has become commonplace and is now considered the norm. When all this cool new technology was introduced, the importance of the natural way of things was completely overlooked – things that people had done instinctively for generations. These natural processes weren't valued and they became lost or, rather, we lost our way. Now there is so much scientific evidence out there to support the fact that things like immediate skin-to-skin, delayed cord clamping and active birthing positions offer numerous benefits to parent and baby. As a result, things are changing and returning to the way they used to be. These things I've just mentioned are now recommended by the National Institute for Health and Care Excellence (NICE) and are considered best practice, based on new findings and updated guidelines. However, they are not innovations at all. For thousands of years people have birthed their babies in upright positions, brought their babies immediately to their chest and not rushed to immediately sever the cord. We used to birth on instinct, but we have been so conditioned through repetitive negative representations of childbirth in the media that we have lost sight of what feels normal and natural.

Take birthing positions, for example. The majority of us still give birth on our backs, despite the fact it is known to be the single worst position to give birth in and increases the risk of requiring an instrumental delivery and tearing. It's also a position that you would not instinctively adopt due to restricted space, going against gravity and so on. It simply doesn't make any sense when you think about it. Yet people choose to give birth on their backs without giving it much thought because they perceive this to be the norm: there is a bed in the room and we are conditioned to lie down on beds, plus, everyone we see giving birth on TV does it this way.

If you feel angry about how common it is to go into birth feeling uninformed and frightened, and you understand how detrimental the fear factor perpetuated by the media is, then the best thing you can do to change the status quo is to tell your friends about hypnobirthing. Shout it from the rooftops! Give them this book and promise them that no fanny whispering or hypnosis is involved. By doing this we can all contribute to changing the way we approach and experience birth.

The good news is that there is definitely a positive shift happening now, and hypnobirthing is a big part of that shift: a return to the natural, instinctive nature of birth and a recognition of the huge benefits this approach brings. Even in theatre, with the rise of gentle caesareans, the way C-sections are routinely done is changing because there is now a recognition of the importance of things such as skin-to-skin, slow birth and so on. A gentle caesarean tries to emulate a vaginal birth as much as possible, including applying pressure to gently ease baby out of the abdominal incision so that the fluid on baby's lungs is squeezed out, which is what happens as a baby moves down the birth canal in a vaginal birth. It's really quite amazing!

Of course, the way things are done in birth is also constantly evolving to meet the needs of those who are expecting. The more informed someone is, the more likely it is that they will request things to be done in a way that best benefits them and their baby. The more frequent the requests become, the more likely it is that common practice will change for the better.

Unfortunately, hypnobirthing can't guarantee you the perfect birth – nothing can promise you that. There are too many variables that no amount of relaxation can control for. However, hypnobirthing *will* equip you with the tools you need to ensure you get the best birth for you on the day.

Hypnobirthing ensures you are informed and empowered to make decisions that feel right for *you* and *your baby*. It will equip you with techniques you can use to remain relaxed and in control throughout, making labour more comfortable and ensuring you meet your baby feeling calm and confident. Ultimately, hypnobirthing practice will help make your birth experience a positive one, however you choose to bring your baby into the world. The benefits of a positive experience are profound and long-lasting.

Wherever you currently are on the anxious-to-excited spectrum, by the time you finish reading this book I want you to feel confident and excited about giving birth, because it's truly the most awesome thing you will ever get to do in your life.

1

The science stuff

Understanding the science behind hypnobirthing is crucial. This is my favourite part of the course to teach, and the part I always cover first, because it brings even the most sceptical on board. I think when people understand *how* the body works and therefore *why* it's so important to be relaxed (so the muscles can work effectively), the more committed they are to the relaxation practice that comes later. Without understanding the all-important how and why, the relaxation techniques taught in hypnobirthing can, admittedly, seem a little fluffy and at worse irrelevant. In this chapter we will cover the physiology of birth: how the muscles of the uterus work when you're in labour, how your hormones can work for and against you, and, most importantly, what you can do to ensure that your birth is as quick, easy and straightforward as possible.

The muscles of the uterus

I suppose the best place to start is with the uterus – your baby's current place of residence! It's the uterus that is going to be working hardest in labour, so it's a good idea to be familiar with it.

When I was pregnant with my second baby and on a hypno-birthing course, I was actually relatively surprised to learn that my uterus – my womb – was simply two bands of muscle. Perhaps I'm in the minority with my poor anatomical knowledge, but I'm willing to confess and accept the potential shame, because maybe, just maybe, it will be a surprise to you too.

I'm not entirely sure what I thought my uterus or womb was. If pressed, I think I would have said the uterus was an organ and there were muscles involved and it grew in pregnancy – a bit like the placenta (another thing I'd given very little thought to). In any case, it transpires that my uterus (and yours!) is just two layers of muscle that stretch in pregnancy to accommodate the growing baby. In labour, the two layers of muscle work in unison, just like so many other muscles in our bodies, to open the cervix and then push the baby out. They are perfectly designed to do this. The more you learn about the uterus, the more amazed you will be. Contrary to the way birth is portrayed in popular culture and the media, the uterus does not have a flaw in its design that has somehow slipped under the radar over millions of years of evolution. No! The uterus will do its job perfectly – if we just allow it to.

So, let me describe how these layers of muscles move in labour. Firstly, there is an inner layer and an outer layer (see opposite). The inner layer is made up of horizontal rings of muscles that are more densely packed towards the bottom of the uterus, because it's these muscles that support the weight of the baby and the waters, holding it all in place. The outer layer is made up of vertical muscles that reach up and around the internal layer.

THE MUSCLES OF THE UTERUS

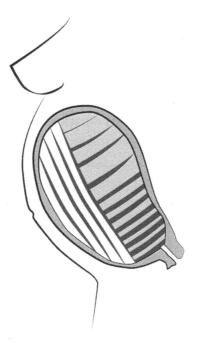

When you are in labour and you experience a contraction or 'surge' (in hypnobirthing we tend to use the word 'surge' because it sounds nicer and more accurately describes the wave-like sensation you will experience), the outer layer of vertical muscles draws up while the internal layer of horizontal muscles remains soft and relaxed. Each time the vertical muscles pull upwards the soft horizontal rings of muscle are slowly gathered up. This continues until you are 10cm dilated. The combination of the muscles moving in this way, and the weight of the baby's head pressing down with each surge, helps the cervix to open (or dilate) to 10cm. This is known as the first stage of labour or the 'up stage' of labour.

Then it's time to get the baby out. The uterus muscles will begin to move in the opposite direction; instead of the outer layer drawing up, the inner layer will now push downwards, easing the baby out. This stage is called the second stage of labour or the 'down stage'. Again, what we see on TV doesn't usually accurately reflect this part of birth. Most often we see people on their back (not an ideal position), red in the face and pushing for their lives, whilst a matronly midwife or doctor stands beside them urging them to push more and push harder. The reality is that your uterus muscles will push your baby out. They are designed to do this and are therefore pretty powerful. The best thing you can do is allow the muscles to do their thing without interfering. Being relaxed is key at this point as tense muscles will not be able to work as well.

What's happening at this stage, on a muscular level, is that the internal rings of muscle that were drawn up during the first stage of labour, and which are now gathered densely at the top of the uterus (the fundus), will start to push downwards with each surge. There's a lot of power in those gathered muscles and sometimes a baby can be ejected pretty quickly.

The cervix

Whilst we are discussing the uterus, it's worth mentioning the cervix. When we talk about 'dilating to 10cm', we are referring to the cervix, which opens to approximately 10cm during the first stage of labour.

So what is the cervix? The cervix is often called 'the neck of the womb'. If you imagine a balloon, the cervix is the knot at the bottom that keeps all the air in. Towards the end of pregnancy, and then even more so during labour, the cervix undergoes some pretty dramatic changes. In early pregnancy your cervix (if you were able to reach it!) would feel firm like the end of your nose. I say *if* you could reach it because the cervix is usually posterior, pointing towards your bottom. Towards the end of pregnancy or in early labour, the cervix starts to move from being a posterior cervix (pointing towards your bum) to aligning with the vagina, so your baby can make their exit. The cervix also softens and begins to feel more like the soft, stretchy part of your earlobe. It then starts to thin (efface) and open (dilate).

A cervix that is thin and soft at the end of pregnancy is often described as a 'ripe' or 'favourable' cervix. One that is still firm and pointing towards your bum is called an 'unfavourable' cervix (which seems pretty harsh in my opinion). But if you hear these words being bandied about, you'll know now what they mean!

One of the most interesting things I've learnt about the cervix is that the changes are initiated by something called fibronectin. This is a protein that the *baby* releases into the waters around it, which is then registered by the cervix, which starts its process of ripening. Mind blown.

If you are thought to be in premature labour you will usually be offered a swab to check for fibronectin. If you're found to have fibronectin in your vaginal fluid it could suggest a preterm labour. However, what's most significant is that if no fibronectin is found, doctors can say with a high level of confidence that you are very unlikely to be going into labour now or for the next two weeks.[1] The release of fetal fibronectin is an essential prerequisite for labour to begin, which means that the happy mantra 'my baby comes when baby is ready' is more than just a positive affirmation; there is some real truth behind it. Remembering this bit of trivia and being able to trust that your baby will come when your baby is ready can really alleviate some of the stress you might experience in the latter weeks of pregnancy as you await your little one's arrival.

U.F.O. positions

What's a flying saucer got to do with anything? Well, just to be clear, I'm not talking about *that* type of U.F.O. and I promise you I'm not about to launch into some strange birth-alien analogy. No, U.F.O. is an important acronym to remember when it comes to giving birth.

U is for UPRIGHT
F is for FORWARD
O is for OPEN

Any position which enables you to be upright, forward and open is the best position for giving birth. Now I'm not going to be prescriptive and tell you that squatting or all-fours is the single best position, because that wouldn't be true. The best position for you is the one that feels most comfortable for you. Everyone's pelvis is slightly different, as is every baby and the position of that baby as they descend. This means that different positions will feel more comfortable for different people. That said, whatever position you adopt, try and remember to be upright, forward and open.

Good U.F.O. positions include: squatting, kneeling, standing, leaning over a table or hospital bed, sitting on a birth ball, sitting on a birth stool, sitting on the toilet and on all fours (see opposite for some examples). I'm pretty sure this list isn't exhaustive! There are many positions which enable you to be upright, forward and open. To clarify, 'upright' doesn't mean you have to be standing straight and tall. *Upright* simply means having gravity on your side, as opposed to lying down. So, kneeling, sitting on a birth ball, squatting – these all count as 'upright' positions.

So why is U.F.O. so important when it comes to giving birth?

U.F.O. POSITIONS

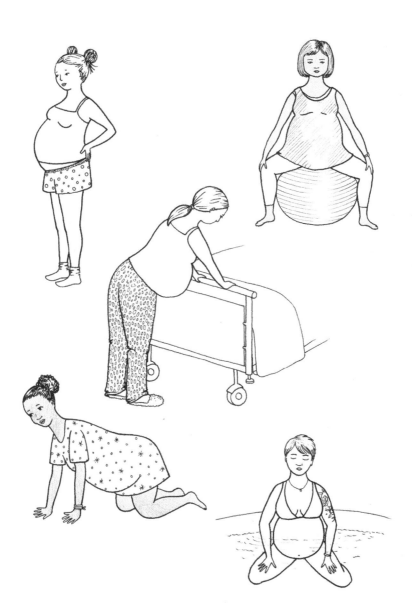

Having gravity on your side helps speed up your labour and birth. When you are upright the weight of your baby's head (the heaviest part of their body) will weigh down on your cervix. This pressure, in combination with the surges, will help your cervix to dilate. Then, when it comes to the down stage of labour, gravity will help your baby to descend down the birth canal as your uterus muscles push powerfully.

Lying down, flat on your back, means you don't have gravity on your side and, although your uterus muscles are strong and powerful, they may not have the power needed to push your baby uphill! That's why the risk of requiring intervention and assistance – in the form of forceps or ventouse to pull the baby out – increases if you are not upright.

Being in a *forward* position, as opposed to being in a reclined position, helps because your baby will be encouraged into the optimum position for birth; head down, back to bump, baby looking towards your bottom.

If you lean forward, gravity will help ensure the back of your baby's head rests by your pubic bone and their back runs parallel with your bump. Whereas if you recline, gravity can pull the back of your baby's head around to your coccyx, so that their back now runs parallel with your own – this is known as a 'back to back' baby. There is nothing wrong with having a back to back baby and babies are born vaginally in this position all the time. It's really very common. But by adopting a forward position when giving birth you're doing what you can to encourage your baby into the optimum position and ensuring a quicker and more comfortable birth for yourself and your baby.

Finally *open*! Obviously, nobody is going to try and give birth with their legs crossed, so what I really mean by 'open' is giving your body the space to open to its full potential. Your body will be full of an amazing hormone called 'relaxin' when you are in labour. In fact, in pregnancy you already have a lot of relaxin in your body. This hormone is responsible for softening all the ligaments, muscles and connective tissue in your body so that everything can stretch to accommodate your growing baby. Quite miraculous really. You may have noticed that your ribcage has expanded and your hips have become wider. All that is down to relaxin – your body is literally making room for the baby!

Now, on the contrary to allowing your body to open, if you lie flat on your back you actually restrict your body's capacity to open by approximately 30 per cent. Your coccyx cannot move and push through a mattress, so it remains in position, and your pelvis is unable to stretch and open as it would do if you were in a U.F.O. position. As a result, the space available is significantly smaller and therefore it becomes more difficult for your baby to be born and the risk of requiring intervention increases.

Knowing all of this, it should come as no surprise that giving birth on your back statistically increases the risk of you experiencing a tear or requiring an episiotomy (where a small cut is made into the perineum in order to open the space), slows down the descent of the baby and increases the likelihood, as I already mentioned, of you requiring assisted delivery (ventouse, forceps). All in all, it's safe to say that being flat on your back is the single worst position for giving birth and the only one I would advocate you avoid.

However, as you probably know yourself, it's the position that seems most common. If you ever see someone give birth on TV (whether it's a film or a documentary or a drama), they're almost always flat on their back. Due to this conditioning by the media, it has become normalised and we have come to accept that this is what birth looks like – that this is a 'normal' position. We desperately need to see more images of people birthing in U.F.O. positions because the current portrayal of birth has damaging consequences; people go into hospitals uninformed and voluntarily lie on beds without thinking. This has many implications for their labour and birth, much of which could be avoided.

But now you've read this, you know! Assume a U.F.O. position wherever you are (home, birth centre, hospital) and it will make the *biggest* difference to your birth.

Your baby's position

Ideally by 36 weeks your baby will be head down and in position. However, some babies don't seem to get this important memo! And if your baby *is* head down, it's possible for them to be 'back to bump' or 'back to back'. So, what do these terms mean? What are the implications? And what can *you* do to encourage your baby into the optimum position for birth?

Back to bump A baby is considered back to bump if their spine runs parallel with your bump. This would usually mean the back of their head is by your pubic bone and they are looking towards your bottom. This position is considered the optimum position for birth.

Back to back A baby is considered back to back if their spine runs parallel with yours. This would usually mean that the back of their head is by your coccyx and they are looking forward. Babies born in this position are sometimes referred to as being born 'sunny side up'. Babies are born this way all the time without a problem – at home, in birth pools, etc. (although it can mean the birth is longer). It's worth knowing that babies can move from 'back to back' to 'back to bump' quite easily and sometimes even do so during labour itself.

It's thought that the reason so many babies are born back to back these days is down to our lifestyle. Those in the generations before us would have spent the majority of their waking hours in a U.F.O. position, tending to small children or doing housework, gardening, farming, etc. There would have been little time to sit down. However, nowadays it's not unusual for us to spend a great majority of our waking hours sitting down. If you want to encourage your baby into the optimum position – back to bump – you will need to be mindful of the positions you regularly spend time in and try to adopt a U.F.O. position whenever possible.

But ultimately, don't worry if your baby isn't in the 'optimum' position. Babies are born back to back all the time. Your labour might be slightly longer and the sensations might feel slightly different (lower back pressure is common) but other than that, there's nothing at all wrong with your baby coming out sunny side up!

Head down or bum down? Prior to 36 weeks it's of little concern which way baby is facing as it's common for babies to move around inside the womb – as I'm sure you are well aware. However, by 36 weeks, midwives like the baby to be head down, as they are less likely to move after this point. If your midwife suspects that baby is bottom down (known as 'breech'), they will refer you for a positioning scan. If the scan confirms baby is breech then there is likely to be some discussion about your options with regard to turning baby and the birth itself.

What muscles need

A lot of what you learn in hypnobirthing, when you actually think about it, is really quite logical and even common sense...

Let's start by asking the question: what do muscles need to work? Not just the uterus but all and any muscles in the body. What do your leg muscles need in order for you to be able to run fast? What do your arm muscles need for you to be able to lift weights?

Muscles need three key things to be able to work effectively and these are oxygen, blood and water. In all instances when you are exercising or doing something physically demanding your muscles need to have a good supply of blood and oxygen in order to function and to be hydrated and fuelled if they are to work effectively. The same goes when you are in labour; essentially you are exercising, as the uterus muscles will be working hard doing their amazing thing.

So, how can we ensure your uterus has a good supply of blood and oxygen and is well hydrated? Well, the last one you can tick off the list pretty easily. The answer is simple: make sure you are having regular drinks throughout your labour. Having a birth partner who knows to offer you sips of water, coconut water or even an energy drink between surges will ensure this happens.

The blood and oxygen are *slightly* more tricky to control but not impossible. The muscles really need oxygen to be able to work and blood is what carries the oxygen to the muscles, making both pretty essential. You can ensure you are taking in lots of lovely oxygen by mastering a good breathing technique.

The direction of the blood flow, however, is not under our direct control so that's where things get a little more complex. To understand the impact a reduction in blood flow can have on a muscle, I want you to try this very short one-minute exercise. I call it the 'timed, elevated-arm, hand-clenching demo'. Catchy, I know!

What I want you to do is lift one arm straight up in the air, above your head. Now quickly clench and unclench your fist, stretching your fingers right out and then clenching your fist each time. This clenching and unclenching is representing the uterus muscles when they are surging. Now I want you to do this for one minute. Within about forty-five seconds, it will be noticeably harder to do, not to mention painful. You will be desperate to stop.

What's happening is that gravity is preventing the blood from reaching the hand as easily as it would if your hand was resting by your side. Because the blood carries the oxygen, this means that not enough oxygen has been able to reach the hand for the muscles to work effectively. The reduction in blood and oxygen to the hand has a dramatic effect – and very quickly: your hand slows down and starts to hurt.

Apply this analogy to your uterus muscles in labour. If the blood supply, and therefore oxygen levels, are reduced, the muscles of the uterus will not be able to work as well. They will slow down and become less effective, making your labour longer. The lack of oxygen reaching the uterus muscles also means it will be more painful, just like it was with your hand. You will very quickly feel the difference.

So it *is* possible to experience real pain in labour, just as you experienced pain in your hand. The good news is that it doesn't have to be like this; there is another way! So long as your uterus has a good supply of blood and oxygen, the muscles will be able to work efficiently and comfortably – as they have been designed to. Labour can be powerful and exhausting – like an intense workout – but it doesn't have to be painful. Pain is usually a signal to your brain to let it know that something isn't quite right; it's an effective method of self-preservation. If you are running on an injury, you will experience pain in the area of the injury and this lets you know that your body isn't ready, but needs time to heal. You then take heed and stop. Similarly, if you have a stone in your shoe you will receive a message to your brain to say; 'Hey! This hurts. You've got to see to this now!' And so you would stop and remove the stone before continuing on your way.

It doesn't make sense that you would send this same message to your brain when in labour. If everything is unfolding as it is meant to, why would you get a message to say 'Something isn't right here and this needs to stop'? It would be completely counterproductive. You don't want labour to stop! You don't want to carry your baby indefinitely. On the contrary, you *want* your baby to born. What's happening is actually completely *right* and there's no reason for it to stop. There's no reason for your brain to receive that pain alert.

The reason someone might experience pain in labour and receive that alert to their brain is if their uterus muscles (and baby) don't have enough oxygen. Pain is the body's way of letting the brain know that something isn't right; the uterus muscles (and baby) need oxygen pronto! Once the person relaxes, the blood and oxygen will be sent to the uterus where they are needed and everything will quickly feel more comfortable.

The obvious question here is *how* can you ensure your blood and oxygen go to the right place in labour? The good news is that when you are in spontaneous labour, the body (because it's clever) will send the blood carrying all the lovely oxygen straight to your uterus (where it's needed). Ensuring it stays this way is another thing altogether though. The solution lies in being relaxed and as your hormones play an important part in this, it's necessary to understand their role.

The hormonal rollercoaster

I'm not talking about pregnancy as a whole (although that too can be a hormonal/emotional rollercoaster), but rather specifically what happens in labour when it comes to your hormones. It's really important that you understand this bit because it's key to having a better birth. Luckily, it's quite simple to get to grips with and very logical.

There are two main hormones you need to know about: oxytocin and adrenaline. Let's take a look at oxytocin first.

Oxytocin

You may have heard of oxytocin before – it's often dubbed the 'love hormone' because you release it when you're in love and when you have sex. You know that giddy, happy, excited feeling you get when you fall in love? When it feels like all is good in the world? That's oxytocin! It's your happy hormone. You also release it when you laugh, when you cuddle, when you're intimate, when you're surrounded by friends and having a great time. Most significantly, you release it when you're relaxed and it makes you feel good. Remember this point because we are going to come back to it. It's an important one.

Oxytocin is produced by the autonomic nervous system, so it's not something you can directly control, but what you *can* do is encourage the production of oxytocin by taking certain steps. For example, you might not be able to flick a magic switch so that your body is full of oxytocin, but you could initiate intimacy with your partner that could lead to foreplay and/or sex and then if you were to orgasm you could be pretty confident that your body would be producing oxytocin. That's what I mean by *encouraging* the production of oxytocin; we know what feels good for us and we can choose to do that. Of course, it doesn't have to be sex – it could be a bubble bath, candles and your favourite music. Whatever it is, you can make a conscious effort to create an environment in which you feel safe, relaxed, loved and happy. This is the environment in which oxytocin flows.

Why is oxytocin so important when it comes to birth? The answer is that oxytocin is actually the hormone responsible for fuelling *every single surge* (contraction) you experience. It's not a 'would be nice to have' item that has the potential to make labour more comfortable; it's an essential ingredient required for labour to get going in the first place. So essential, in fact, that if you opt for an induction, the drug you will be given is syntocinon, which is simply a synthetic version of oxytocin.

I've already mentioned a few examples of when you might release oxytocin, namely situations in which you are relaxed and feeling good. Sex is often given as an example because when you orgasm your body releases a whole load of it. That's why an orgasm feels so good! I also said to remember that point about needing to be relaxed to produce it and it making you feel good ... now, consider birth ... are you beginning to join the dots?

Mind-blowing game-changer fact

Labour is *designed* to feel good!

Your labour is fuelled by oxytocin – *fact*! Oxytocin makes you feel good – *fact*! Labour can feel good – *fact*! You release oxytocin when you feel happy, relaxed and safe. Which is exactly how you need to feel in birth too.

Once you understand the role of oxytocin, you understand why relaxation is key to making birth a lot easier. All of the relaxation techniques we teach in hypnobirthing are motivated by this simple fact: we need oxytocin to fuel our surges (contractions) and we need to be relaxed in order to produce oxytocin. Hence, we need to learn how to properly relax in pregnancy so that we can access this feeling and state of being when it comes to birth.

So, if the hormone that at all other points in our life makes us feel fantastic is the same hormone that we produce in labour, why do we grow up thinking birth is going to be horrible and painful - something we need to 'get through', a necessary evil, a trauma even. Why do we think it is something to be feared when it is designed to feel good? And it truly is. At the moment of birth your body will have the highest level of oxytocin in it – more than any orgasm previously experienced – and you will feel bloody amazing! Birth, when you are relaxed and everything is going well, can feel good. Intense, like a workout, but good.

Oxytocin ensures that the uterus surges and also signals to your body that you are relaxed and all is well, so that the blood carrying the oxygen is directed to the uterus muscles (and the baby) where it is needed. Labour then progresses quickly and efficiently and, although it can be hard going at times and exhausting, you will feel good and strong. Soon you will be holding your baby in your arms and feeling like a superhero. That is how birth is designed to happen.

Now for the second hormone that you need to know about: adrenaline. I'm pretty sure you will have heard of this one, but let's look at it more closely.

Adrenaline

Adrenaline is the hormone your body releases when it perceives some sort of threat. The threat doesn't even have to be real – a *perceived* threat is enough to trigger the release of adrenaline. The body takes no chances. It could be that you had a near miss in the car or even a full-blown near-death experience, but equally you might just be watching something scary on the TV and are beginning to tense up, breathing more heavily as your heart beats that bit quicker: you bet that any minute now the killer is going to jump out on the main protagonist. Even if you *know* it's just TV, your body still goes through the same motions.

Like oxytocin, adrenaline is produced by the autonomic nervous system, so it's something that happens instinctively and not something you can directly control. That's the bad news. The good news is that, just like with the oxytocin, you can take steps to discourage (rather than encourage) the production of adrenaline and also take steps to lessen the impact if you do produce it. It all comes back to mastering the relaxation techniques that are commonly associated with hypnobirthing.

If you were to plot adrenaline and oxytocin on some sort of hormonal spectrum, they would sit at opposite ends. Whereas oxytocin is all about happiness and relaxation and feeling good, adrenaline is all about panic, fear and the grisly fight for survival. Basically, as far away from feeling relaxed as is possible.

So, when you release adrenaline, what happens? Your heart rate speeds up and you experience that heart-pounding sensation. The heart is working extra hard and super-fast to pump the blood around your body. It's being pumped somewhere specific and the clue is in the phrase used to describe this mode you're in: 'fight or flight'.

Your heart is pumping your blood as fast as it can to your arms and legs, so that you can fight, if need be, or run (take flight) from the threat. It's the body's life-saving mechanism and, in many situations, it can actually be life-saving ... if there is a need to be super-strong or super-fast. However, when giving birth it's not terribly helpful; in fact, I'd go as far as saying it's terribly *un*helpful.

The blood, which is full of lovely and very vital oxygen, is being redirected *away* from the uterus and sent to the arms and legs. Now your limbs might at this point become super-strong, fully charged with copious amounts of oxygen, but it's not these you need to birth a baby! Your uterus, which is still trying to do its job, is now being deprived of the oxygen it requires to be able to work at full capacity and is beginning to struggle and slow. If you recall the exercise we did earlier with the fist clenching, that same thing is now happening with your uterus muscles. The blood supply and oxygen levels have been reduced and now the uterus muscles are feeling the effects.

Just like when your hand was elevated in the air, the muscles of the uterus will become more painful and slow down, making each surge (contraction) less effective. This means that your labour will become longer as progress (dilation) will slow.

Another unhelpful, but relatively obvious-when-we-think-about-it thing that happens when adrenaline is released, is that it inhibits the production of oxytocin. It's not possible to simultaneously feel relaxed and happy *and* fearful and panicked. Imagine for a moment that you are at home, lying on the sofa watching something funny on TV and then suddenly you hear a loud crash upstairs. What happens? You don't slowly transition from feeling relaxed to becoming alarmed; it's instantaneous. You are immediately on high alert, your heart pounding and your body flooded with adrenaline. Moving from one state to another can happen incredibly quickly and anything can set us off. It doesn't even have to be a trigger as explicit as a loud crash. It could be an evocative smell that reminds you of a time when you felt scared or distressed. It could be a snippet of conversation you overhear between a midwife and a doctor about another patient. It could be recalling something you saw on the news or read about, or a traumatic birth story someone once told you. Any of these things could trigger the release of adrenaline, which then immediately inhibits your oxytocin – your feel-good factor.

A reduction in oxytocin will result in your surges becoming less effective (since oxytocin is fuelling them) and dilation will slow down, again making your labour longer and increasing the risk of/need for intervention.

You can now understand why some people might experience long labours, describing it as being very painful and not reflecting very fondly on their birth experience. The more adrenaline you have in your body through feeling frightened, the longer and more painful your labour will be. You're a lot more likely to require intervention to help speed things up, and pain relief to cope. Your baby is also more likely to experience distress as they tire due to the longer labour, and also due to the reduction in blood flow and oxygen. Your body is a clever thing and it will always prioritise saving your life over your baby's. Your uterus might be doing wonderful and miraculous things in growing new life, but the uterus cannot save your life, so if there is a threat (real or perceived), the body will take the blood and oxygen away from the uterus and send them to the arms and legs, where it believes they are needed in order to fight or flee the imminent danger that threatens your life. It's not quite clever enough to recognise that the 'threat' may not be real and that you're not going to thank it for depriving your uterus and your baby of vital oxygen when your life doesn't actually need saving. Once you understand how the system is designed to work, it's clear that being frightened about birth does nobody any favours.

Interestingly this isn't new knowledge! In fact, the negative impact fear has on birth was recognised some time ago by a famous British obstetrician called Dr Dick-Read. He explored the knock-on effect of fear back in the early 1900s and developed a concept which is now known as the fear, tension and pain cycle.[2]

If you feel anxious and frightened in labour, the blood and oxygen going to the uterus muscles are reduced and thus the muscles become more tense and then more painful (remember the clenching fist). If you are experiencing increasing pain, do you think you would feel more or less frightened as time goes on? More frightened of course! And then the cycle continues and the panic mounts: fear results in muscle tension and pain, and the pain causes the fear to increase and so on and so on.

This is sadly a common scenario that can unfold: someone is in labour and feeling frightened and producing adrenaline. Their uterus muscles will still be trying to do their job, but with limited blood and oxygen they will be struggling; the person in turn will be experiencing increasing amounts of pain. They will start panicking. They will probably be examined and told that they have not progressed (because the uterus muscles aren't able to work effectively). The pain is getting worse, but there is still no progress. So they will feel more panicked, not knowing how much longer they can take it. Their baby is likely to start showing signs of distress, which in turn is likely to increase their panic and pain, and so now they're calling for pain relief as it's too much to handle. Now there are doctors in the room, they are talking about pain relief and how to speed things up as their baby isn't coping well with the labour and they are not progressing. They have a few options – they could be hooked up to a drip to speed things up using artificial oxytocin and then perhaps an instrumental delivery, or they could have a caesarean section.

It's scary, but also understandable how things can unfold in this way, and how quickly a pathway in birth can change once someone is producing adrenaline. You are probably nodding along right now, because perhaps you have experienced the above in your own previous labour, or heard stories from friends and family; the above is hopefully helping you make sense of what you have been told. It all stems from feeling fearful about birth, which is very, very sad, but, with focused effort and commitment, fear can be overcome.

I'm not saying intervention is entirely avoidable because there are variables in pregnancy and birth that no amount of relaxation can negate, but the feelings of fear and the ensuing panic are. Being calm will put you in the best position to navigate your birth, however it pans out. It is true in every single case: the more relaxed you are, the better your birth will be.

Fear → Tension → Pain

When it comes to the initial fear that sets this cycle off, it could be a fear about labour and birth, a fear of pain or a fear of being in hospital. All lead to feelings of anxiety, stress and panic and the production of adrenaline.

The person then starts to experience pain, because the muscles send a message to the brain to say something is wrong and needs to stop. It's not the labour that's wrong and it certainly doesn't need to stop! The thing that's wrong is that the uterus muscles don't have enough oxygen to work properly. That's why it feels painful. That's why the person's brain is receiving a warning alert and they feel pain. The more painful it becomes, the more the person starts to panic, thus producing more adrenaline and so enabling this negative cycle to continue.

But do not worry, we are going to *break the cycle*. We are going to do this by removing the fear and equipping you with practical tools that you can use to remain calm and relaxed throughout birth. If you are calm in your mind and relaxed in your body, you won't produce adrenaline and therefore you won't experience increasing amounts of pain. In fact, quite the opposite: your labour will be more efficient, quick and comfortable.

Even if you have a little wobble in labour, the good news is that adrenaline leaves the body quickly, so as long as you don't *keep* producing it, it's possible to move back into a calm and relaxed state, enabling the oxytocin to flow once more. The techniques you will learn in this book will help you do just this. So, if you do have a slight panic, don't worry. It's not game over! It's never game over.

2

The toolkit

It's time now to get to grips with the amazing and life-changing hypnobirthing toolkit. In this chapter I will take you through the two breathing techniques (game changers, the pair of them), some visualisations, light-touch massage, guided relaxations, positive affirmations and the art of creating shortcuts to relaxation. Enjoy.

And breathe ...

Breathing is the single most important thing you can do in labour. If you take nothing else from this book, take this!

A good breathing technique helps you in many ways; firstly, it ensures you are bringing oxygen into your body which, as you know, your muscles need to be able to work effectively. You wouldn't try to exercise whilst holding your breath. Same goes for labour and birth. Secondly, by remaining committed to a breathing technique you are ensuring that you remain relaxed and avoid panic breathing/hyperventilating. Finally, by focusing on your breath through each surge, you are redirecting your focus away from the sensation you are experiencing, which makes each surge more manageable. Instead of being swept up in the waves and feeling out of control, by sticking with your breath you are remaining calm and grounded. The counting that goes alongside the breathing technique or the visualisations can be hugely helpful in keeping you on track.

In this chapter you will learn two very simple and easy breathing techniques. These alone will transform your labour for the better and I don't say that lightly! I recommend practising them as much as possible so that they become second nature. The first breathing technique, which I call 'up breathing', is a lovely calming breath and you can use it throughout the day to bring some relaxation into your life. Certainly a few rounds of this breath before bed will help you get to sleep. The other breathing technique, which I call 'down breathing', is a great one to use when going for a poo. So, the toilet is the perfect place to practise this one! To help, at the back of this book you'll find a practice schedule which you can use if you wish. How much you practise is, of course, up to you, but the more practice you put in, the more effective all of these tools and techniques will be.

To keep things super-simple, up breathing is for the 'up stage' of labour, where the muscles draw up and the cervix opens. Down breathing is for the 'down stage' of labour, where the muscles begin to move downwards, gently pushing the baby out.

The first thing I want to reassure you about is that you *will* know when you've entered the down stage and it's time to change your breathing style, because you will feel your body beginning to push and you will feel your baby moving down the birth canal; it's an unmissable sensation. It doesn't matter if you're a first-time parent-to-be, trust me; you will know. It's a bit like doing a poo. How do you know when you need to go? You don't wait until the poo is halfway out before going to the toilet (at least, I hope you don't!). You usually experience a feeling of pressure beforehand and you just know.

The second thing I want you to know is that there is no need to worry about what might happen if you forget to switch and continue to use your up breathing throughout the down stage of labour. The answer is absolutely nothing bad will happen. If you're happy breathing in for four and breathing out for eight throughout your entire labour and birth, then that is absolutely fine; the most important thing is that you keep breathing! As long as you are bringing in oxygen and breathing out rather than tensing and holding your breath, you are doing an amazing job and it will be profoundly more comfortable.

However, what you might notice is that when your body starts to push it will become more difficult to continue with the up breathing. It's hard to inhale slowly and feel your chest rise and expand as your uterus muscles push downwards in the opposite direction. You might notice that you start to make a mooing sound as you exhale, as your body simultaneously and involuntarily pushes downwards powerfully. Again, this is totally fine and indeed very normal – it might just indicate that it's time to switch to down breathing, which will be a lot easier to do at this point.

Up breathing

This is the most important one to master as it's the one you'll most likely use for the longest amount of time. Nobody can tell you how long your labour will last (sorry!), but a general rule of thumb is that the first stage, the 'up stage', where the uterus muscles draw up and the cervix softens and opens to fully dilated, is longer than the second stage, the 'down stage', in which the uterus muscles change direction and push the baby down the birth canal and out into the big wide world. This stage can last anything from a few minutes to a couple of hours, whereas the first stage is likely to last several hours (although, of course, not always).

The good news is that up breathing is very easy to do and also feels really nice, so it's a breath you will hopefully *enjoy* practising.

It's also worth noting that this breathing technique is not a hypnobirthing-specific one. It is used to help people suffering from insomnia and anxiety, and is also used in mindfulness practice. It's effective because it slows the heart rate and helps you to relax; it really is a skill for life.

So, let's give it a go!

Make sure you're sitting comfortably. In a moment I want you to close your eyes to block out what's going on around you. Then I want you to inhale deeply through your nose, filling your lungs, whilst slowly counting to four. Then I want you to slowly exhale through your mouth, allowing the air to slowly pass through your lips, whilst counting to eight.

At first you may find it tricky exhaling for eight counts, especially when pregnant, since the baby inhibits your lungs from filling to their full capacity. However, it will get easier through practice, and when you're in labour and your baby moves further down into your pelvis, you will find you are better able to breathe. If you're really struggling, try exhaling for a count of six instead. Just make sure your exhale is longer than your inhale; this will feel calming and relaxing. This breathing technique is the opposite of panic breathing or hyperventilating, where someone inhales faster and faster and their exhale becomes shorter and shorter and almost non-existent. We are aiming for the opposite effect.

Let's try now . . .

Breathing in, 2, 3, 4 and breathing out, 2, 3, 4, 5, 6, 7, 8.

Now I want you to do the same again, but this time doing four repetitions of the breath. So in for four and out for eight, four times over. If you have someone with you, ask them to count for you.

Ideally, you're now feeling nice and relaxed. It's normal to feel a little light-headed. In fact, the more you do this breath, the more you'll feel like you are floating on a little cloud. It's a bit like natural gas and air, and most people really enjoy this feeling.

The reason I asked you to do the up breathing four times over is significant. Four repetitions of the up-breathing technique takes about forty-eight seconds. This is how long a surge or contraction generally lasts when you are in established labour. Imagine a surge (contraction) slowly building to a peak of intensity, before easing off and releasing until you feel nothing at all; if you do four repetitions, the surge will either have passed completely, or at the very least be on the release – you will have got over the peak.

Thinking of surges in this way, breaking it down, really helps to make labour more manageable. Lots of people hear stories of labours lasting hours and have this idea that, once labour starts, it's one long contraction until the moment of birth. The reality is that you will experience a surge, lasting about forty-five seconds to a minute, then a little break of a few minutes and then another surge. This is the pattern that established labour generally follows; three surges in a ten-minute period, each surge lasting about forty-five seconds. This pattern may well last many hours but broken down in this way and dealt with surge-by-surge makes it a lot easier to handle.

Milli Hill once calculated that during a regular labour, you only experience any sensation at all for approximately 23 per cent of the time.[3] The other 77 per cent of the time, you experience nothing at all. So even if your labour is ten hours in total, you will only be experiencing the sensations of labour for just over two hours.

I love the affirmation 'every surge brings me closer to my baby'. There are no wasted surges. Deal with each one as it comes; close your eyes, begin to inhale, count to four, then slowly exhale and count to eight. Do this four times over and by the time you finish, the surge will have passed and you know you are another step closer to meeting your baby.

Another favourite affirmation of mine is 'inhale peace and exhale tension'. I imagine my body expanding and filling with peace as I inhale for four and then, as I exhale for eight, I imagine all tension releasing as my whole body softens and relaxes. I hope you will enjoy practising this breathing technique and use it not just for birth but for life, in times of stress. It's a very simple but incredible powerful tool you have. Best of all, you have it with you always and it's completely free. You never need to remember to pack it! You carry your breath with you wherever you go, so don't forget to use it.

Down breathing

At some point your uterus muscles will start to push downwards and you will feel the change in direction, and then the mounting pressure as your baby descends. This is the time to switch your breathing technique.

This stage is less about relaxation (although it's always important to be relaxed) but is more active; you are birthing your baby! I use the analogy of blowing out a candle; you wouldn't slowly exhale as the flame would just waver and not go out. You would direct your breath with purpose. You would use your breath with intent. This is what happens with down breathing; you use your breath with focus and intent. As you exhale through your mouth, you channel your breath downwards to help your muscles push your baby down and out.

There is no counting involved when it comes to the down stage of labour. You simply take a quick, big breath in through the nose, filling your lungs and then as you exhale through your mouth, you channel that out breath down through your body. And then you repeat. And you do this until the surge has passed, at which point you can return to your normal breathing.

I appreciate most people find the up breathing easier to master; you inhale for a count of four through your nose and you exhale for a count of eight through your mouth – easy peasy! Down breathing without the counting, on the other hand, is a little trickier to get your head around. To help you, I have a few tips and tricks.

As you practise down breathing, rest your hands just above your hips, at the bottom of your ribs. As you inhale you will feel little movement but as you exhale, if you're exhaling with focus and intent, channelling your breath downwards, you should feel your muscles respond and almost push downwards with your breath. Try it a few times. If you feel your muscles move downwards with your breath, you know you've cracked it. During the down stage of labour your muscles will be pushing downwards powerfully with each surge and by using this breath you are ensuring that you are working with your uterus muscles rather than against them. You are helping to make everything more effective. You are not pushing, you are using your breath to help your muscles. It's your muscles that will be doing all the hard work.

When it comes to practice, down breathing is not one that is going to help you drift off to sleep peacefully, which is why I always recommend doing your practice in a particular place, or should I say when doing a particular 'activity'.

Yes – on the toilet when going for a poo! It's the perfect time and place to practise your down breathing. I always suggest you stick a little sticky note on the back of your toilet door at home and simply write 'down breathing' on it as a little reminder. Then when you go to the toilet, let's say once a day, you're ensuring regular practice. Not only that, but you're beginning to condition yourself to associate the down-breathing technique with relaxing and softening, and with something being expelled from the body. Yes, it's a poo, rather than a baby, but that sensation of mounting pressure does feel pretty similar to that at the beginning of the down stage of labour. You might even find the down breathing helps you go for a poo – more breathing, less straining! Either way, the more you practise, the more it will be second nature to you on the big day.

You might also find it helpful when watching positive birth videos on YouTube to listen in extra carefully towards the end, just before the baby is born. Try and tune in to see if you can hear the person in the video using their breath in the down stage of labour. This might give you a good idea of how down breathing is used in practice.

Finally, it's common to worry about how you will know when you have entered this down stage, but you really will just *know*. You will feel your body begin to push downwards and it's an unmistakable sensation. Lots of people I've taught have said that at this point they naturally switched to down breathing because it felt more comfortable to do – it wasn't a conscious decision.

Visualisations

Some people will really love the counting technique for breathing and will come to rely on their birth partner to count for them, coaching them through each surge. If this works for you, then that's brilliant. Practise with your birth partner – it's a great way for them to be involved. Other people might prefer the room to be quiet or to listen to music or relaxation readings.

If you don't find the counting relaxing or you don't have someone to count for you, then another way to pace your breathing is to use a visualisation. It's a good idea to use an upward visualisation to accompany your up breathing. For example, you might like to imagine a hot air balloon: as you inhale, the balloon fills with air, inflating until it's a big round balloon. Then, as you slowly exhale, imagine the hot air balloon gently rising up into the sky and drifting off into the distance.

You might prefer to imagine the sun rising over the horizon as you inhale, then, as you exhale slowly, picture it moving upwards to its midday position above your head. Imagine feeling the warmth of the sun as it rises upwards.

Alternatively, you might like to imagine a party balloon inflating and expanding as you inhale, and then, as you exhale, feel all the air releasing as the balloon shrinks quickly in size. Choose a colour for your balloon as this will help you with your visualisation.

For down breathing, people tend to use opening visualisations. For example, as you exhale you could imagine all the layers of a rose bud unfolding and opening.

Some will use visualisations with which they are already familiar – from yoga classes for example. A common one is the 'golden thread' visualisation: as you exhale you picture a golden thread running from your lips and extending out towards the horizon. If you break your breath you break the thread, an image that might help you remain committed to that longer exhale.

Others during the down stage of labour will visualise their baby moving down the birth canal and focus on the fact they will be meeting their baby very, very soon. Perhaps they will consider what their baby's face might look like or perhaps they will imagine the moment they introduce their baby to siblings or other family members. It's nice to allow yourself to be distracted by these happy thoughts.

It's really a case of whatever works for you and helps you to maintain the in-for-four and out-for-eight rhythm of the breath.

Whatever you choose is fine. Just take some time each day to practise the breathing whilst using a visualisation. Doing a few repetitions each evening before you go to bed is ideal as it will help you relax into sleep, but do also practise whenever you think of it during the day.

At first you will probably find that you still count silently in your head whilst breathing and trying to follow the visualisation. After a bit of practice, you will get used to the rhythm of the breath and what four and eight counts feels like, and will be able to pace yourself, focusing on your visualisation without counting. Practice really is key. Even if you plan on having your birth partner count for you, it's a good idea to also have a back-up visualisation you can use if your birth partner is having to talk to a midwife or doctor, or if you pop out of the room to go to the toilet. You can never have too many tools at your disposal.

Positive reinforcement

In psychology there's something called positive reprogramming, which means rewiring your brain and changing the way you think. The aim of positive reinforcement is essentially the same. However, I think the latter sounds friendlier and less like you're a piece of computer software that's about to be plugged in and rebooted!

Positive reinforcement is simply the act of consciously seeking out positive thoughts over and over again until you change on a neurological level the patterns in your brain (the reprogramming element). Numerous studies have shown that using positive affirmations regularly (listening to or reading positive statements) or engaging in cognitive behavioural therapy (CBT) is effective and changes the way your brain lights up and processes information in your subconscious mind. Amazing stuff.

When it comes to birth, many people feel understandably terrified. No doubt a lot of that fear is down to the media, what we see on TV and the horror stories we hear. However, through positive reinforcement it's possible to replace our negative associations with birth with more positive ones, and, as a result, feel more positive and confident when thinking about birth.

Easy ways that you can start using positive reinforcement to change your mindset include:

- **Listening** to positive affirmations on MP3
- **Creating** or buying a set of positive affirmation cards to place around your home so that you see and absorb positive statements daily
- **Watching** positive birth videos
- **Reading** positive birth stories
- **Looking** at positive birth photography

Here are some positive affirmations to get you started. Repeat them to yourself as often as possible. There are also loads more great resources at the back of the book, so make sure to check them out too.

Positive affirmations

I make decisions that feel right for me and my baby
I love and respect my pregnant body
Giving birth is the most wonderful and empowering experience
I feel calm, relaxed and at ease
My body knows how to nourish and grow my baby
I trust my body is perfectly designed to birth my baby

I will birth my baby comfortably, calmly and confidently
Where my mind leads my body follows
Relaxing my mind relaxes my muscles
The birth of my baby will be beautiful
My baby knows when and how to be born
My baby will come when my baby is ready
My baby is the perfect size for my body
As labour progresses I become more deeply relaxed
I listen to my body and do what it needs me to do
I inhale peace and exhale tension
My birth partner is by my side and on my side
Every surge brings me closer to meeting my baby
My surges cannot be stronger than me because they are me
I am a strong and capable person
All the strength I need is within me
Birth is a safe and wonderful experience
I trust in the instinctive nature of birth
My baby will be born gently, calmly and safely
My job is simply to relax and allow my body to birth my baby
Giving birth is powerful but so am I
I look forward to holding my baby in my arms
I welcome my baby with love and confidence

As important as it is to absorb positivity and build new positive associations with birth, it's equally important to protect yourself from negativity, which only undermines your efforts. Avoid TV shows that you know show dramatic – and traumatic – portrayals of birth, don't be sucked in by clickbait on the internet which you know will lead only to scary or worrying stories, avoid TV dramas or novels that could trigger fear, and have the confidence to ask those who feel it appropriate to share their birth trauma with you at this time to please refrain from doing so – or at least wait until you have had your baby! Try not to absorb someone else's negative experience in the name of being polite, as it will only impact your own.

When I'm teaching I often use the analogy of a filing cabinet. Your brain is full of files and the ones at the front are the easiest to reach and pull out. In pregnancy you want to fill your brain with positive files. These could be positive birth stories, positive birth images, positive affirmations, so that when you're in labour your subconscious mind draws upon the content in these files and you feel reassured. What you don't want is for your cabinet – or subconscious – to be full of negative files, because when you're in labour these are the files your subconscious will draw upon and they will make you feel frightened, which will negatively impact the progression of your labour.

So, go out there and fill that cabinet with positive files and positivity and don't allow yourself to store any new negativity. You've probably had a lifetime of creating negative associations about birth. Now is the time to start building positive ones.

You may sometimes become aware that your mind has drifted and you're thinking of something that concerns you or makes you feel worried or anxious. It may be something you heard in passing, something that apparently happened to a friend of a friend, something you saw on TV or even your own previous experience of giving birth. If this happens, consciously steer your mind back to something positive: read a positive story, watch a positive video, scroll a birth photography account, listen to your positive affirmations. The more you do this, the sooner it will happen that, when you think of birth, or someone mentions birth, immediately a positive thought is triggered.

Positive reinforcement takes some commitment, but the impact is profound and, as with a lot of these techniques, the benefits are felt immediately. By listening to positive affirmations or reading positive affirmation cards you will begin to feel less anxious and more confident about birth right away.

Learning to switch off

It is not typically part of our culture to practise relaxation. Most people, if asked, will say they *do* something to relax – be that running, reading a book, going for a drink or watching telly. We frequently substitute a less enjoyable activity (work, for instance) with a more enjoyable activity (a hobby, for example) and count this as an example of us 'relaxing'. But really, we're merely engaging in a different *type* of activity. We rarely actually switch off and take time out to truly relax.

We all love to distract ourselves from the day's worries and demands by engaging in something more fun. That's not a bad thing at all and it does make you feel good, *but* it's not relaxation practice.

In labour we want to be thoroughly relaxed – in mind *and* body. We know there is a mind–body connection, so if we can achieve a sense of calm in our minds, it makes sense that our bodies will also be relaxed, making birth so much easier.

In hypnobirthing we have various ways of achieving this relaxation. A lot of it might be new to you, but through practice it can become second nature, and, over time, you will find it easier and easier to tap into the relaxed state you are able to create. It's a valuable skill to have for life generally, not just in pregnancy, because regular relaxation offers so many mental and physical health benefits. In some schools, mindfulness and relaxation exercises are being taught to young children as part of the curriculum. Hopefully, the next generation will grow up knowing how to properly relax and able to recognise the benefits of such practice. Even if it's not something you've done before, it's relatively easy (with a little practice) to achieve a state of deep relaxation using some simple tools. And that's what we're going to look at in this chapter.

Guided relaxation exercises

These can also be called guided meditations and are essentially mindfulness exercises. They are about being present in the moment, allowing your mind to be guided by the voice of your birth partner or a recording, and achieving a state of relaxation. This is *not* about being hypnotised or being out of control. During a guided relaxation you are very much *in* control.

I've provided pregnancy-specific scripts for you to use at the back of this book (see pages 219–227). They are designed to help you feel confident about your upcoming birth, and can be read by your birth partner. I've also included links for free MP3s, which you can download, in the Resources section at the back of this book. With the MP3s, all you need to do is find a quiet space, pop your headphones in and play them. Allow your eyes to close when prompted to do so and simply listen to my voice as it guides you through the relaxation exercise.

Although the MP3s can be very effective, it's a good idea to try doing some guided relaxation practice with your birth partner. Their voice is even better as it's already familiar to you and a source of reassurance and comfort. Doing the practice together also helps your birth partner to feel involved. If you want to give this a go, use the scripts at the back of the book. I recommend playing some gentle background music whilst your birth partner reads the script. It might also be a good idea to light a candle, spritz the room with a scented room spray, dim the lights – and add anything else you plan on doing when giving birth. Essentially practise setting the scene! Then ensure you are comfortable (sitting or lying down), close your eyes and allow yourself to be guided through the relaxation by your birth partner's voice.

It may feel funny the first couple of times you do this, but, with practice, it will become routine and hopefully you will find you actually enjoy taking five minutes out of your day to do this exercise together.

Setting anchors

An anchor in hypnotherapy is simply something that you strongly associate with a happy memory. It can be a smell or a particular sound (a piece of music for example), a visual, a taste (a particular food) or a familiar touch.

Another term for setting anchors is 'conditioning'. There was a famous study done in the 1890s/early 1900s known as 'Pavlov's Dogs', which was all about this concept. A scientist, Pavlov, used a metronome to produce a clicking noise and would then feed his dogs. After some time, he discovered that when the dogs heard the metronome they would salivate in anticipation of the food. The food no longer needed to be present to trigger this reaction; the dogs were conditioned to associate the *sound* of the metronome with their food. In this way Pavlov proved that animals – including humans – could be conditioned, through repeated and reinforced association, to respond to set triggers.

When it comes to doing your hypnobirthing practice you are essentially doing the same thing: conditioning yourself to relax in response to certain triggers – be that audio, touch, etc. You are building positive associations now in pregnancy between these triggers and a sense of deep relaxation. Then, when in labour, your body will respond in kind to these triggers. The more you practise, the more powerful and effective the triggers will be.

You'll notice that the first guided relaxation script (at the back of this book) is very simple and your birth partner only needs to read it through and that is all. The following two scripts have a little more going on: the first includes some arm stroking and the second an arm drop – these are two ways that we can set anchors that will trigger relaxation during birth.

Arm stroking

With arm stroking, your birth partner will simply need to stroke your arm slowly, starting at the knuckles, over the hand and up the arm towards the elbow, whilst reading the script. It can be a very light stroke, almost tickly, or a firmer stroke; it comes down to personal preference. By doing this each time the script is read, you will begin to associate the arm stroking with the lovely, deep relaxation you are hopefully experiencing. Then, when in labour, your birth partner may not have time to read the whole script, but they can use the arm-stroking element. This will be a trigger for you and help to ease you into that lovely, familiar, relaxed state. Hypnotherapists call this 'setting an anchor'. In this case, the touch is the anchor and you associate it with the deep relaxation you have experienced when practising at home, feeling safe and comfortable. I like to think of it as creating a shortcut to relaxation.

It's worth knowing this works for anything else too! If you prefer having your hair stroked, you could ask your birth partner to do this instead. It's not that the arm has any special powers, but more that you build an association, through practice, between an action (arm stroking) and a feeling (relaxation). You can then use the action as a standalone to trigger that same feeling in labour.

Arm drops

The second script includes an arm drop. When prompted to do so within the script, your birth partner needs to gently take hold of your wrist and raise your arm a little above your lap. If it's properly relaxed your arm should feel heavy to lift. Then, when prompted to do so within the script, your birth partner will release their hold on your wrist and allow your arm to drop into your lap. If you have remained relaxed your arm should be limp and heavy, falling without resistance. If your arm hovers and appears to defy gravity this would suggest you are holding onto some tension in your body and are partially lifting the weight of your arm yourself. By repeating this arm drop three times, you will be encouraged to really let go and release all tension.

Of course, a limp, relaxed arm is not directly going to make birth easier, but if your arm is limp and relaxed, the chances are that your entire body is also free of tension. The more relaxed the muscles are throughout your body, the more comfortable your labour will be, and the easier it will be for the baby to descend and be born, because there is no resistance or internal struggle. On the other hand, if you are holding onto tension in your arm, your core is likely to also be tense and drawing up. This will make the descent of baby more difficult as the muscles draw up and hold your baby in.

As with the arm stroking, the more you practise, the more effective this exercise will be. The more familiar it is, the faster your body will respond, recognising that when your birth part-ner takes your wrist to raise your arm you are to hand over the weight of your arm to your birth partner and let go of any ten-sion. It can work powerfully at the right time and, as with the arm stroking, can be used as a standalone trigger for relaxation, as well as being used within the context of the relaxation script.

A lot of our behaviour is conditioned without us even being

consciously aware of it. As humans we are very receptive to patterns and routine, so aim to incorporate your relaxation practice within your normal daily routine and it will soon become second nature. For example, you could aim to set aside some time each evening before bed to practise relaxation. Before bed is a particularly good time to practise because you should feel nice and relaxed and well ready for sleep by the time you've finished the exercises. The practice also offers immediate benefits so it shouldn't feel like an arduous chore; rather, I hope it's something you'll look forward to doing each evening because it's enjoyable and feels good and will soon become as routine as brushing your teeth.

If you take a moment just now to reflect, you can probably identify a number of things in your own life that you already do which trigger a certain response. These triggers could be sounds or smells, or they might help us feel awake or help us go to sleep, or make us feel happy or sad, energised or hungry. For example, for me, putting on my slippers immediately signals that I'm at home and relaxing rather than going out and being busy. For others it might be soaking in a bath, a certain scented candle, a foot rub. If there is something you regularly do at home to relax, use that as part of your birth preparation. It will be powerful because you've already been doing it for years. You don't need to build a new association if one already exists. You just need to find ways of incorporating into your birth what you already do at home to relax.

Always remember that the end goal is to be relaxed in mind and body. How you get there is less important. The important thing is that you get there! Try out some of the suggestions in this book, try some of the things you already do, and cumulatively you will find you have a toolbox full of things you can use in labour.

Light-touch massage

The word 'massage' here is slightly misleading as this technique is more about the light *touch* than massage in the traditional sense. This is not deep-tissue massage and there's no working of the thumbs deep into the muscle. Instead, your birth partner will use the backs of their fingertips to lightly stroke your back, trailing their fingers slowly and lightly against your skin.

So, birth partners – you should always start with both hands at the base of the spine, just above the coccyx. You then move your hands up the spine, backs of the fingertips in light contact with the skin, before branching out as if you are drawing the lower layers of a palm tree's leaves. Begin again at the bottom, this time going up a little further and then again, branching out and letting the backs of your fingertips trail lightly as you bring your hands back down. Start again at the bottom, going a little higher this time before branching out, around and down. Continue until you are reaching the base of their neck before branching out across the tops of their shoulders (see the illustration overleaf). Then begin the exercise again at the bottom and repeat it over and over. Always keep the touch light and move slowly and gently. Visualise drawing a palm tree on their back as you go.

It may feel repetitive or as if you're not doing much at all, but hopefully the lucky recipient will be experiencing a lovely tingly feeling spreading out throughout their body – this is the oxytocin. By stimulating the nerve endings of the spine you're encouraging the production of not only oxytocin but also endorphins. Endorphins are the body's natural pain relief and are believed to be many times stronger than morphine. Endorphins stick around in the body and make you feel good,

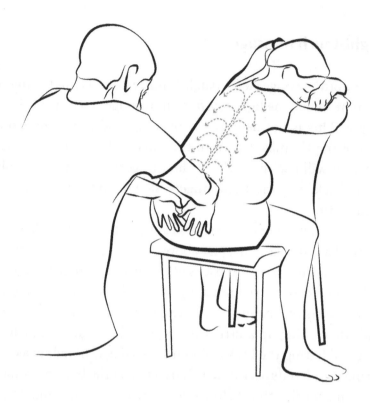

so the more of these the better.

Light-touch massage works in a similar way to a TENS machine (Transcutaneous Electrical Nerve Stimulation). A TENS machine has four sticky pads that are placed on your lower back, and these are attached by wires to a small, handheld device. A rhythmic electrical pulse is then emitted and you can control the strength of it – turning it up or down. The device usually comes with a boost button that you press when experiencing a surge. When you press the boost button the rhythm changes and a different sensation radiates throughout your back. It takes some getting used to initially, but after a short while you almost won't notice it. The way it works in terms of pain relief is that the electric pulse stimulates the nerves into producing endorphins, just as light-touch massage does.

You can buy a TENS machine especially for labour and birth from pharmacies, or you can hire them from various places. Your midwife should be able to advise. You want one suitable for pregnancy because there are other types available for those suffering from back pain that work in the same way but might not be suitable for use in pregnancy.

Light-touch massage is a personal favourite of mine and it's something birth partners can do *between* surges to help the person in labour to relax and produce more of the good, happy hormones. The TENS machine is also useful for this and it can be used at home in early labour, as well as when labour is more established. The only place you can't use a TENS machine is in a birth pool, for obvious reasons! Other benefits of the TENS machine is that nothing passes to baby, like a drug might, and if you don't like it you don't have to wait for it to leave your system, but can simply switch it off. Whether you choose to use light-touch massage or a TENS machine, or a bit of both, is totally down to personal preference.

By now you should start to feel like you have a good toolkit coming together ready for birth. I always recommend giving each exercise a fair try, even if at first it seems a little funny or ineffective. These may well be new skills you are learning and not something you have ever done before, so it could take a little time to get to grips with them or warm to them. However, if you have tried something a number of times and it's really not aiding your relaxation then let that one go and focus on the techniques that *do* work for you. As long as you have a few tools you can rely on to help you relax, that's great. Never lose sight of the main aim of the game: to be relaxed. How you get there doesn't really matter. You might use an arm drop, you might not. You might use something entirely different. You might choose to customise your toolkit with techniques you already employ to help you relax. What matters is that you get there. I hope that at least some of these techniques will help you achieve that wonderful state of relaxation.

The breathing techniques, along with the counting or visualisations, are certainly the most important to master and should be used during each surge. The light-touch massage, guided relaxations, arm-stroking and arm-drop techniques can be used between surges to help you deepen your relaxation and let go of any tension acquired during the surge.

When it comes to practising, I have included a practice schedule at the back of the book for you to use if you wish. I would recommend setting aside time each day to practise. It doesn't have to be a lot of time! Maybe ten or fifteen minutes. You don't need to practise every single technique every single evening. I'd recommend starting your practice with a few repetitions of the up breathing to slow things down and get you in the mood and then doing one of the guided relaxations *or* the light-touch massage. Then pop your MP3s on or play some relaxing music of your choice as you drift off to sleep. If you do this each evening, you will be very well prepared.

BIRTH STORY

Home water birth – Antonia, second-time parent

This was my second home birth, with our first child being born on the sofa two years previously. Although my first labour was technically 'good' with no complications, I certainly felt it was traumatic and struggled to cope with the intensity at times. I realised looking back that I hadn't really believed in my ability to birth my baby, so when push came to shove (quite literally) I panicked and ended up leaving the birth pool and pushing whilst being coached by others. I remembered feeling totally out of control and, although proud I'd managed to give birth at home, a bit traumatised by the whole thing. In fact, the first thought I had when they placed Solly into my arms was 'I am never doing that again!'

This is why, when Sam and I found out we were expecting our second child, I knew so much I wanted to conquer this fear and make my next birth something I could be really proud of. With some practice and positive thinking I was truly able to change my mindset about labour, and started to (dare I say it) look forward to the challenge!

On the day of my labour I woke up at 1.30am with what felt like the start of contractions. I immediately went into a minor default panic but knew that if I could just stay in bed and conserve my energy I would be helping myself out massively. I started listening to my relaxation track for hypnobirthing and breathed through all the feelings I was having until they started to come with some frequency. When we finally called the midwife in the morning I felt calm and relaxed. By 8am I was in established labour. Sam and I were in the lounge together, candles burning, music playing and very much in our own space.

When things started to hot up, and I got into the pool, Sam helped me remember my breathing. This helped massively: him knowing what I needed made me feel like we were in it together. Also, for Sam, I think it made him feel much more included than in my first labour when he perhaps felt like more of a spectator.

I remember so many of the affirmations going through my head when I felt overwhelmed and them really calming me down. In particular, I found comfort in the fact that I was not alone and *that parents all over the world were doing this with me. Instead of in my first labour when all I wanted was for the surges to stop, I almost welcomed them as I knew they were bringing me closer to my baby.*

Finally, and most miraculously for me, was the fact that I got to believe in myself and my ability to trust my body and birth my baby vaginally. My midwife was amazing and in those final surges simply stood back and allowed me to birth my baby. I literally couldn't believe what I was feeling: my baby coming to me naturally without any need to be told to push. The reflex was so strong and within a couple of big surges he came floating up between my legs to meet me.

To say it was amazing was an understatement. This birth was such a gift and has left me on a high I don't think I'll ever come down from. For anyone who is nervous or may not trust in their ability, I could not recommend hypnobirthing enough. If only all parents had access to it, the way we think and feel about labour and birth would be different. I am forever grateful for my chance to own my birth instead of being overwhelmed by it. There really is no greater gift!

3

Talking sense

We have established by now how important it is to feel relaxed when it comes to birth. In a nutshell: the more relaxed you are, the more oxytocin you will produce. Not only does this hormone speed up labour and make for an easier birth, it also reduces blood loss after birth, helps establish breastfeeding, aids bonding and reduces the risk of postnatal depression. Being relaxed also feels good (bonus) and by being relaxed in your body on a muscular level, you're allowing everything to soften, open and release, as intended.

As we've discussed, the opposite happens if you are feeling anxious and scared: you produce adrenaline and your body enters fight-or-flight mode, which means your blood (carrying all that lovely and much-needed oxygen) is redirected to your arms and legs and *away* from the uterus muscles. This causes the uterus muscles to become *less* efficient and *more* painful, and progress slows – and can even stall (not so good). With blood and oxygen to the uterus reduced, baby is more likely to experience distress, which of course causes someone in labour to panic even more; thus more adrenaline is produced and they enter the horrible cycle of fear → tension → pain.

So, we can all agree that the aim of the labour game is to

remain as relaxed as possible throughout. We've talked about how relaxation exercises can help, but another simple thing you can do is address the environment you find yourself in.

Being at home is ideal *if* it is the right choice for you: it's already a (hopefully) relaxing and familiar environment. However, for a whole host of reasons, home might not be an option or, indeed, where you feel safe or most relaxed. But all is not lost – far from it! The good news is that *wherever* you plan to give birth (theatre included) there is a lot you can do to create a space that feels calm, safe and familiar.

I use this word 'safe' a lot. The reason being that if we *feel* safe, we tend to relax. Whereas if we feel threatened it's unlikely that we'll be able to relax. Therefore, choosing a place to give birth and creating a space in which you *feel safe* is key.

Feeling uninhibited is also important when it comes to giving birth because it enables you to fully relax and go with the flow. Therefore consider how the environment (and the people in it) will affect how you feel: usually if you're aware you are being observed (by strangers especially) and feel under scrutiny or pressure, or are in a brightly lit space, you will feel more self-conscious and inhibited. This is why it's *very* important to give careful thought to how you want your birthing space to be, and who you want in it!

So, what can you do to make even the most clinical of spaces feel safe, calm and familiar?

It all comes down to our senses! We 'read' our environment, the space around us, through our five senses: sight, smell, sound, taste and touch. We often absorb all this information without being consciously aware of it, yet it informs how we feel in any given space, at any time.

In order to transform a space into an oasis of calm and tranquility, we simply need to ensure each of our five senses is met with something that brings us comfort and helps us to relax.

In labour our senses are often heightened, which means *everything* you do to bring relaxation and comfort will be even more powerful.

Using the five senses as a simple checklist, I want you to take a moment to consider what you would like to see, hear, smell, taste and touch that would help you feel calm, safe and relaxed.

Sight

What would you like the space to look like? What would you like to *see* to help you feel more relaxed? The majority of people will prefer to have low lighting. It is well known that you will feel more relaxed and less inhibited or self-conscious with the lights turned down. The good news is that most birth centres (and even some labour wards) offer dimmable lighting. But, in any case, I recommend getting yourself a small box of battery-operated tea lights just to make sure you have a way of controlling the lighting. Once switched on in a dark room they look pretty realistic (despite being plastic). The reason I recommend battery-operated ones over real ones is that you can't have an open flame in a hospital or birth centre. And even if you're planning a home birth, it's good to have them as a back-up, just in case you do transfer in or your candles burn out.

Fairy lights are another alternative, but the great thing about battery-operated tea lights is that you don't need access to an electrical socket for them to work, and most people will associate candlelight with romantic, intimate occasions – where, generally, they will have been relaxed and producing oxytocin!

Other things you might like to see are familiar items, perhaps photos of your older children if you have them, or some positive affirmation cards which you might like to place around the room.

Whatever it is, as long as it helps you feel relaxed and calm, then it's a good choice.

Smell

Smell is hugely evocative and the slightest hint of a fragrance can conjure up long-forgotten memories. It's powerful stuff.

When it comes to birth, we want to harness this power and use it, as we've said many times now, to bring relaxation and comfort. You certainly don't want to be smelling the distinctive smell of a hospital or cleaning products – or anything else less savoury for that matter!

Essential oils are great, especially ones such as lavender and camomile, which are well known to aid relaxation. (*Be careful, though: some essential oils are not recommended for use during pregnancy, so be sure to check this out before using them.*)

You can always buy yourself a room spray with essential oils in it or put them in a diffuser or oil burner if at home. Or you may already have a favourite scented candle which you light to help you relax. Room sprays are great because they are very portable, as are rollerballs, which you can use to safely apply essential oils to your pulse points, like a perfume.

Many room sprays that use essential oils can smell like a luxury spa. Most people will associate that spa-like smell with relaxation and positive, happy thoughts (even if they've not had many spa breaks!), so something like this would be perfect.

Whatever you choose to do, make sure you have a way of making the space smell nice with a scent that conjures up happy memories of relaxed times. Giving a room a quick spritz is a very easy and quick way to transform the feeling of a space. When you have your eyes closed and you're breathing deeply it will work wonders.

Sound

What do you want to *hear* when you're in labour? Do you want to hear people talking about their weekend plans or what they're doing after work? Do you want to be aware of the hustle and bustle going on around you? Conversations between other parents and medical professionals? Probably not . . . Remember, what will help you *deepen* your relaxation?

For a lot of people, it will be music, so a good idea would be to prepare a playlist with a mix of upbeat, happy tunes and calmer, relaxing music. Favourite songs will often conjure up happy memories so be sure to include these. Music, like a scent, can be very powerful and transport you to another place and time. Make sure it's a good place and time!

Other people will enjoy listening to guided relaxations or positive affirmations, especially if they have listened to these tracks during their pregnancy. The audio will be very familiar and hearing it in labour will be comforting.

Others might choose to use generic background music, for example spa music. With your eyes closed and the combination of gentle pan-pipe music playing and the smell of essential oils filling the room, you could almost believe you were on a spa break! All these things might seem little on their own, but collectively they can make a *big* difference to how relaxed you feel.

Of course, you might listen to all of the above when in labour – alternating between your favourite songs, positive affirmations, guided relaxations and spa music. Just make sure you have the tracks loaded onto your phone or other device ready to play, and pack in your birth bag either a small portable speaker or a set of headphones (or both) so you can listen on the big day.

Taste

What can you eat to bring you comfort and make you feel happy? What might you look forward to opening when it comes to the big day? Remember, labour is a lot like a workout – those uterus muscles will be working hard for quite some time – so it's important to fuel up and ensure you're well hydrated throughout. You wouldn't run a marathon on empty, would you?

So, pack lots of drinks – water, coconut water, maybe a can of something fizzy – and also non-perishable foods that you might like to snack on when in labour. Make sure you pack yourself a treat – if there was ever a time for a little reward, it is most definitely now!

> **TOP TIP** Whilst we're on the topic of food and drink, make sure your birth partner has supplies packed for himself/herself as well. Nothing worse than a hangry birth partner!

Touch

What can you wear that you will feel comfortable in? Think about fabrics that are cool or cosy, depending on the time of the year. Think about the clothes you usually wear when you want to feel relaxed. Consider what you might want to wear if you use a birth pool – a bikini top perhaps?

Remember the most important thing is that you feel comfortable, relaxed, unrestricted and ideally not self-conscious. Avoid wearing a hospital gown if you can, as this will send the message to your own mind that you are a patient and that something is wrong, because generally those are the associations we have with hospital gowns and they are deeply embedded within our subconscious. One might be offered to you if you are admitted to hospital, but you can always choose to wear your own clothes.

You might like to wear a dressing gown and slippers, a simple oversized cotton T-shirt, some baggy tracksuit bottoms, your PJs or even a summer dress. The choice is entirely yours.

You might also like to consider packing your own pillow or perhaps a blanket – anything that helps you feel *more* relaxed and comfortable. Familiar items are especially good as you have so many positive associations already established with them.

Don't forget massage oil. This would fall under touch. Many massage oils contain essential oils that are safe for pregnancy and can aid relaxation. You might opt for one of those or you might prefer to use a tub of pure coconut oil. Coconut oil is great for massage and also super moisturising for the skin – as well as carrying associations with piña coladas, thanks to the coconutty smell! Anything that reminds us of cocktails (or mocktails) on sunny summer holidays is probably a good thing.

So there we have it. Sight, Sound, Smell, Taste and Touch: the five senses and an easy checklist for you to use to ensure you are a creating a space that is conducive for birth, a space that feels calm and safe and enables you to fully let go and relax.

The great thing about this checklist is that it makes it *so* easy to transform a space. And best of all, it can be used wherever you are: be that at home, in a birth centre or on a labour ward. Wherever you find yourself, as long as you have the bits and pieces with you in a birth bag, you can, in a matter of minutes, change the entire mood of a room. Flip the light switch, lay your candles out, spritz your room spray, get the playlist going, wear your comfies and soak it all up whilst sipping on coconut water and munching on jelly babies! Even the most clinical of spaces can be transformed into an intimate and romantic spa-like space.

Even if you birth your baby in theatre, possibly the most clinical space there is, you *still* have the power to change the space so that you can meet your baby feeling calm, safe and relaxed. Always go back to the five senses and think what you would like to see, smell, hear, taste and touch. In theatre you can ask for the lights to be turned off and the surgeon to use a spotlight to illuminate the area where they will be working. This means that once baby is born, they can be lifted up on to your chest and be immediately in a darker environment, which will be far less alarming. You might even be able to place some of your battery-operated tea lights around your head, so you feel as if you're in a candlelit space. You can also choose to have your music playing in theatre, or positive affirmations or any other MP3s. Again, this can help you to feel more relaxed. You might like to use a roller-ball with essential oils that aid relaxation on your pulse points. You might bring in your own pillow or blanket. You wouldn't be able to eat or drink in theatre and you probably wouldn't be wearing your comfies, but there is still lots you can do to change the external environment – and that will have a significant and positive impact on how you feel in the space.

Do make sure you give some due thought to the above and how you will create the perfect space for *your* birth. Collect all the items needed and pack them in a birth bag ahead of time, whether you're planning a home birth or not, so that everything you need on the big day is easily accessible together in one place. It will make life a LOT easier. Finally, make sure your birth partner knows what they are to do, as it's likely to fall on them to set the scene. You'll find a birth-bag packing list at the back of this book, which might prove useful here.

Remember: set the scene for the birth *you* want!

If you're someone who feels particularly anxious about birth and you still feel sceptical as to whether the tools you have learnt will really help you on the big day, Gemma's experience will hopefully reassure you.

Birth Story

Gemma, a first-time parent who had her baby
in the birth pool at her local birth centre

I had always feared childbirth from a young age, due to being
so scared of needles. I faint at the sight of blood and hospitals
just make me anxious. But I knew I needed to overcome all this if
I was going to fulfil my dream of becoming a mum – the only title
in the world that I've always wanted. I thought I would try hypnobirthing as an option to keep me as calm as possible. I practised
my breathing and spent evenings going over the affirmations.

I went eleven days over my 'estimated due date' and tried
many of the suggested things to kick-start labour – curries,
lavender oil, walking, lots of stairs. My mum, whom I wanted to
be my birthing partner alongside my husband, finally came to
stay and on the Sunday evening we had a lovely bbq in my back
garden, which must have got that oxytocin flowing!

By 9pm I had dull period pains on the sofa, which continued
throughout the night, although completely bearable, making me
question if this was really it or not. I managed to sleep through
a lot of them.

I went for a walk in the morning with my husband and by 11am
the surges were getting a little more intense. I had my exercise
ball, and my breathing techniques and used both of these until
4pm when the surges were getting three to four minutes apart.
We called the birthing unit and they said to come in for a check.
Mum, my husband and I could not believe it when I got to the
midwife-led birthing unit and they confirmed I was 5cm dilated

and would be staying in. The midwives also couldn't believe how calm I was. I used my breathing techniques and got in the zone. My mum made the room look lovely, sprayed lavender spray, and I had my favourite drinks and food on hand. The midwives even gave me an aromatherapy hand massage. It was like being in a spa – exactly the atmosphere I wanted! I now needed a little gas and air to help me along, though, as the surges were getting quite intense, but not painful. I thought of every single one as a step closer to meeting my baby boy.

When the surges got more intense and I was 8cm dilated, I asked to go in the water. Wow. It felt amazing. I knew instantly that this was where I wanted to have the baby, although I had been unsure on the run-up. I could not believe I was about to give birth. I felt calm, relaxed and in control – not what I was expecting all those years leading up to it! Then my body told me it was time. I was quite tired by this point, but my birthing partners kept me focused. It was time to change to down breathing, and within around ten pushes my baby was there in the water. I lifted him to my chest – my precious baby boy! Everyone in the room was crying with tears of joy.

Who would have thought that the girl who couldn't handle a blood test in October could birth such a chunky baby on gas and air, water and breathing techniques? I still can't quite believe it.

4

Choosing where to give birth

Do not for one moment underestimate the impact your choice of birth place will have on your birth. Spoiler: it's huge! We may have learnt how to transform even the most clinical environment into a tranquil, spa-like space, but in terms of decisions that need to be made pre-birth, choosing *where* you plan to give birth is up there as one of the most important decisions you will make in your pregnancy.

When you first see your GP in your pregnancy, you are generally referred for a booking appointment at your nearest hospital. Or perhaps you have gone straight to your local hospital and arranged a booking appointment directly. Either way, it's important to realise that you are not limited to your nearest hospital. You can in fact 'shop around' and, if you want a hospital or birth-centre birth, choose the one that is best for you. In fact, that's the case for all NHS care: you don't need to be seen at your nearest hospital. If there is a specialist hospital elsewhere in the country, you can request to be referred there. You actually have a lot of say in the matter! It's not a postcode lottery.

So how do you decide where is best? Firstly, the internet is your friend here. Lots of hospitals and birth centres have virtual tours available, so visiting their websites and seeing what's on offer is a good place to start. Some hospitals and birth centres might offer you the opportunity to visit in person too (it's always worth phoning ahead to see if this is possible). If this is an option, it's worth taking for a number of reasons. Firstly, it's good to do a practice run (drive) and learn your way around the hospital/birth centre. These places are often like mazes, so knowing where you need to head in advance of the big day is really useful. Secondly, by visiting in person, the place becomes that bit more familiar, which means you will feel more relaxed when you arrive to give birth.

You may want to look up the hospitals and birth centres that are near you and compare what they offer and see how their birth outcomes measure up against the national averages. For example, things like what percentage of people give birth in water, require stitches, and have an unplanned caesarean or birth without any intervention. You might also want to find out what is on offer – for example, different types of pain relief, birthing stools, bean bags, dimmable lighting, etc. Knowing what's available might help you to make your decision, but it also helps you plan for what the space is going to look like and what you might need to bring from home.

A resource that I would recommend looking at, especially if you're a stat fan like me, is the Birthplace Study.[5] The study, conducted in 2012, evaluated the birth outcomes of 64,000 women in the UK, so there was a huge cohort. All the women were considered 'low-risk', meaning they had no known medical issues that would suggest complications were more likely.

The study compared the birth outcomes for parent and baby in four different settings: obstetric units (traditional labour wards), freestanding midwifery units (standalone midwife-led birth centres), alongside midwifery units (midwife-led units on hospital grounds) and home. The findings were *very* interesting.

The case for home births

Giving birth at home can be a truly wonderful experience – one without the hassle of having to navigate a journey to hospital or anywhere else, as midwives come out to you and are in a position to give you their full attention. You often enjoy continuity of care, meaning the same midwife or group of midwives will see you at all of your antenatal appointments, your birth and your postpartum visits. There is also the sheer bliss of being able to get into your own bed after giving birth and snuggle up with your newborn baby. All that said, one of the most common reasons people dismiss home as an option is because of the big 'what if?' question (which is essentially based on fear): 'What if something were to go wrong?' And if you've ever been in a situation where you've told someone you are considering a home birth, no doubt your news will at some point have been greeted with the loaded remark: 'You're brave!' That implies you are doing something risky and dangerous, when the thing is, for a lot of people, it's not brave at all; it's a sensible choice and the best place for them. The problem is that we, as a society, are so conditioned to believe birth is dangerous and hospital is the safest place. In reality, intervention rates are much higher in hospitals, even for for those considered 'low-risk', which actually raises the question: 'But what if something goes wrong in hospital?' What if the reason something is going wrong is *because* you are in hospital? The truth is, nobody should have to justify their birth-place choice; it's your choice and nobody else's. And there's no right or wrong choice either. What's most important is that every expectant parent understands their options and is able to make a properly informed choice, and not one based on fear or conditioning.

One of the most significant findings from the Birthplace Study was that for a 'low-risk' second-time (or subsequent) parent, home was the safest place to give birth statistically.[6] That's right! If you are having your second or subsequent baby, and are enjoying an uncomplicated pregnancy with no known medical issues (i.e. considered 'low-risk'), then home is statistically the safest place for you to give birth, with no significant difference in outcome for the baby compared to hospital but with significantly fewer interventions, making it better for both you and your baby.

Interventions include augmentation of labour (using drugs to speed things up), assisted delivery (forceps or ventouse to get the baby out), stitches for trauma (vaginal tears), episiotomies (an incision to the perineum) and caesarean sections. The likelihood of any of these becoming necessary is significantly reduced if you choose to birth at home. Yet, despite the findings of this study being publicly available (perhaps not promoted well enough), the home birth rate across the UK remains at around 2 per cent.

Whilst the above applies to those having their second or subsequent baby, this does not mean that home is not safe if you are considered 'low-risk' and having your first baby. The study showed that for first-time parents the risk of the baby experiencing an adverse outcome, although still very low, increased from 5 in 1000 in an obstetric unit to 9 in 1000 within the home birth group. However, the risk of intervention for first-time parents was still lowest at home. The study also found that those giving birth for the first time were more likely to be transferred to a hospital – 45 per cent compared to 12 per cent of those giving birth for the second (or subsequent) time.[7]

This does not mean that 45 per cent experienced an emergency at home though. Common reasons for transfer include: wanting more substantial pain relief (an epidural), not dilating as quickly as expected, meconium in the baby's waters, or other signs that would indicate continuous monitoring might be a good idea. So, whilst the study certainly doesn't rule out home birth for first-time parents (there are clear benefits as well as risks) it highlights how choosing where to give birth is not always straightforward but requires some careful consideration, research and weighing up of pros and cons. Ultimately, where you choose to give birth has to be right for you; it's your choice.

With regard to the big 'But what if something goes wrong?' question and the common 'I would rather be in hospital, just in case ...' remark – these comments are tricky to navigate, because there's no doubt that if something is *going wrong* you probably would want to be in hospital! But it's a little more complex than simply choosing to be in hospital because it would be the right place to be *if* something went wrong, when, by being in the hospital setting, you're increasing the chances of something going wrong in the first place. It's certainly not clear cut.

By taking yourself to hospital 'just in case', you're immediately increasing your risk of requiring intervention. Essentially, you are increasing your risk of requiring forceps or ventouse, needing a caesarean, having a tear and requiring stitches or having an episiotomy, to name just a few! All because you want to be in 'the right place' in case something goes wrong. But a lot of what might go wrong could potentially be avoided – and certainly the risk significantly reduced – by not being in hospital in the first place, and in fact being somewhere better suited to giving birth.

So, before you rule out home, I'd like to make a couple of points – food for thought, if you will.

Firstly, when you are having a home birth, you will have one dedicated midwife with you throughout your labour and a second one who will join you closer to the point of your giving birth. You therefore have wonderful one-to-one care with a midwife who you are more likely to know because you will have had your antenatal appointments with this home-birth/community team. Having a midwife with you whilst you are in labour, focused solely on you and your baby, is far better than being in a busy hospital where you might find yourself sharing a midwife with another parent. At home you will have the full attention of a midwife who will give you support and closely monitor you, so that if there was any reason for concern you could transfer into a hospital and be attended to at the earliest opportunity.

Secondly, midwives are not risk-takers, especially not midwives supporting people birthing at home, knowing they do not have easy access to a back-up medical team. Midwives, quite literally, have your and your baby's life in their hands and that's a big responsibility. If your midwife thinks that you or your baby might need some support, they will recommend you make the transfer into hospital. They will not wait until an emergency has unfolded before recommending going in. Hence the transfer rate – they don't take risks.

Thirdly, calculate the time it would take to transfer into your nearest hospital by ambulance (with blue lights) and compare that to the average time it takes to transfer from a hospital ward to theatre in an emergency situation. If there is not much difference, then that should reassure you considerably. It is worth knowing that, even if you are in hospital, there is no guarantee that a theatre will be empty and a team ready and waiting for you. Often they will have to bring people in who are on call, or clear the theatre and prep for you, which takes time. If you are transferring in from home the paramedics will have called ahead and all of this will be happening whilst you are travelling in, so that by the time you arrive you can go straight in and be seen by the appropriate person.

Mind-blowing game-changer fact

For second-time (or subsequent), low-risk parents, home is the *safest* place to give birth statistically, with the best outcomes for parents and babies and the fewest interventions.[8]

BIRTH STORY

Home water birth after trauma –
Eshere, a second-time parent

After a traumatic long labour with an episiotomy and ventouse with our first child I can happily say hypnobirthing changed our lives!

My second baby was born in the birth pool at home in under three hours with no pain relief or intervention and no stitches! A completely different experience to our first birth!

I was extremely nervous and worried about the birth as my first labour was so difficult; however, after doing the hypnobirthing course we felt more informed and embarked on some serious preparation.

After a long day of light surges my waters finally broke around 10.30pm. The surges came in fast and intense. Having a slight panic in my own head, as the surges were extremely intense, my husband Tom reminded me of my breathing and

I managed to stay calm and focused. The midwives arrived pretty quickly and advised me to get in the pool to ensure baby arrived in the water as we planned. The room was perfectly lit with candles, my affirmations playing on our stereo in the background and the pool ready for action. As soon as I entered the water I felt a soothing sensation. I breathed through each surge as I had been practising in the weeks leading up to the birth and felt my baby move through my birthing canal. It was a truly unique and wonderful feeling that I will never forget. During the transition period I felt for baby's head and remember talking with Tom and having an intense feeling of excitement that our baby was coming! With a few more surges our baby entered this world. We really did it!

The case for birth centres

Birth centres are a fantastic middle ground between home and hospital and the recommended birth-place choice for low-risk first-time parents. You can get freestanding birth centres or 'alongside' birth centres which are attached to hospitals. Birth centres are midwife-led and are designed to support vaginal birth with low lighting, birth pools and a calm, private environment. Each birth centre has its own set of guidelines as to who it can accommodate. These guidelines are flexible and it is possible (with a little persuasion and support from a supervisor of midwives) to be accommodated, even if you fall outside the guidelines.

There are no doctors working within a birth centre and also no epidurals available (these require an anaesthetist). Many interventions cannot take place in a birth centre and should they become necessary would mean a transfer to a labour ward, just as with home birth. In fact, what's available in a birth centre is not so different to what's available at home. A birth centre may have more apparatus, such as birthing stools or birth balls, which you may not have at home, but otherwise they are the same: same midwives, same training, same care and same medical equipment.

It's worth pointing out that interventions (for example, caesarean sections) not being available at home or in birth centres is not the reason that intervention rates show as being lower in these settings – the results aren't reflective of what's available at each setting, they reflect the final outcome. In the Birthplace Study, if someone planned to give birth at home or in a birth centre and then went into hospital for an intervention, that intervention was recorded against their original birth-place choice, that being home or birth centre. Hence, when the study shows that there is a 2.8 per cent chance of needing a caesarean if having a home birth, this is not suggesting that 2.8 per cent are having a caesarean at home! Rather, this is the percentage of people who originally intended to have a home birth, but ended up needing to transfer into hospital for a caesarean.

The study proves that the need for intervention is significantly less if planning a home birth or using a birth centre. For example, the risk of requiring a caesarean is 2.8 per cent for someone low-risk planning a home birth, rising to 3.5 per cent if using a freestanding birth centre, and 4.4 per cent if using an alongside birth centre. The risk for the same low-risk person increases to 11.1 per cent if planning to give birth on the labour ward. That's a significant increase and given that a caesarean is major surgery, certainly something to be mindful of when making your choice.

When choosing between home and a birth centre, given that they are quite similar, it might be worth considering things like pets or other children and what your plan would be for them whilst you are in labour, as well as the distance you are from hospital when at home or in a birth centre. Perhaps your home is closer to the hospital than your local freestanding birth centre. Or perhaps your home is quite far from the hospital, but the hospital has a birth centre on site. Transfer time is definitely worth taking into consideration. It might also be worth thinking about how important it is to you to have the use of a pool (home is the only place where you can guarantee yourself an available pool) and also where you feel safest and most relaxed.

If you have a birth centre locally that is attached to a main hospital then you have the added reassurance of being on site should you need extra assistance. This might make you feel more relaxed.

Although you will need to take into account travelling into a birth centre when in labour, the plus side is that once there you don't have to do much else in the way of admin; a midwife will take charge of sorting the birth pool and you won't feel you have to do any hosting. The down side is that a pool is subject to availability and sometimes birth centres can get full, meaning you can't be accommodated and would need to go to the labour ward.

Ultimately, if you are considered to be 'low-risk' and you choose to use a birth centre you can be happy knowing you're significantly reducing your risk of needing intervention and improving your overall birth outcomes in comparison to going to hospital.

The case for hospitals

If you're under consultant care and don't fall within the 'low-risk' bracket, chances are you will have been recommended to give birth in hospital on the labour ward. This does not mean this is your only option (although you may have been made to feel this way). The first thing worth knowing is that you can *always* have a home birth – it is your right. Nobody can come to your home and forcibly drag you into hospital against your will. Now I'm not saying that home is necessarily the right choice for you. I'm just saying you always have the right to be supported at home and so you have that one in your back pocket, so to speak.

Birth centres, as I mentioned before, have guidelines as to who can use them. These guidelines vary from birth centre to birth centre and can be flexible. Depending on the reason you're under consultant care, it is possible in some circumstances to be approved to use a birth centre even though you fall outside the guidelines. You need to speak to a senior midwife and request what's known as an 'out of guidelines care plan' to be created.

There are many reasons why you might be under consultant care but it's important to remember that 'risks' that have been identified are on a spectrum. Some people under consultant care will be easily accommodated and supported in birth centres, while for others hospital will be the most appropriate place.

If the latter applies to you, you still have options. You will have been referred at your booking appointment to your nearest hospital and now be under its care. You have the right, however, to choose to go to any hospital in the UK. I'm not advocating you travel hundreds of miles to get to the hospital of your choice, but do explore the ones in your local area to find the one best suited to you.

You might find that there is little between the hospitals in your area but there could be a significant difference which would sway your decision. For example, one hospital might have several birth pools on the labour ward, and if you want a water birth this would give you more chance of achieving one than in a hospital where only one pool is available. Or perhaps you know you will be staying in hospital for a short while and one hospital doesn't permit birth partners to stay outside visiting hours, while another does. This fact could help you to make up your mind. So, shop around! You don't get to give birth very often in life, so choose carefully.

Know that if you choose hospital because it feels like the right place for you, then it *is* the right place for you. Don't be disheartened by the Birthplace Study if you're under consultant care, because the study only looked at those considered 'low-risk', meaning these statistics don't apply to you if you fall outside this category. If you have an existing medical issue, pregnancy-related illness or some other identified risk factor, then hospital could well be the best place for you. The good news is that there is lots you can do to transform a hospital room into a space that feels as cosy and comfortable as home, and by the time you finish this book you will also have your fail-safe toolkit at your disposal to help you remain calm and relaxed throughout the experience.

Lastly, another resource available to help you make your choice as to where to give birth is the NICE guidelines. The NICE guidelines are evidence-based and produced by the National Institute for Health and Care Excellence and are regularly updated as and when new evidence comes to light. What's also helpful to know is that the NICE guidelines don't just exist for maternity services but for all health services. The NICE guidelines govern best practice within the NHS and so the advice or recommendations made by your local trust should be in line with these guidelines. You can always search the NICE guidelines online to see what the latest recommendations are for the management and treatment of any medical issue you might experience. And if you're ever in any doubt that what you're being told is correct, a quick google of the NICE guidelines will let you know whether or not the advice you're being given is up to date as well as help you understand the reasons behind the recommendations that you have been given.

In relation to choosing where to give birth, the NICE guidelines advise that people are informed that they may choose to give birth in any birth setting and be supported in their choice, that anyone considered low-risk and having their second or subsequent baby should be advised that planning to give birth at home or in a birth centre is particularly suitable for them because 'the rate of interventions is lower and the outcome for the baby is no different compared with an obstetric unit', and that low-risk first-time parents should be advised that planning to give birth at a birth centre is particularly suitable for them because 'the rate of interventions is lower and the outcome for the baby is no different compared to an obstetric unit'. The guidelines also advise that anyone low-risk and giving birth for the first time should be informed that if they plan to have their baby at home 'there is a small increase in the risk of an adverse outcome for the baby'.[10]

If you're reading this and you have no known medical issues, then the statistics should speak for themselves: you can see it's worth at least considering your home or a birth centre as viable options, instead of a hospital labour ward.

It's all about challenging the ingrained assumptions we have that include hospital being the 'right' place to have a baby. The hospital is the right place to have your baby only if you have known medical issues and are likely to need the additional support and assistance that is available there, as well as a specialist consultant's expertise and input. If you have no medical issues then the stats are in your favour for choosing to birth elsewhere and being cared for by a midwife, an expert in facilitating and supporting vaginal birth.

I believe there are two key reasons why so many people choose to give birth in hospital compared to a birth centre or at home. Firstly, we have been taught to believe birth is a risky and dangerous activity that involves high levels of drama and that people's lives are on the line (thanks, TV). Secondly, many believe birth will be horrifically painful and assume that they'll need *all* the drugs going. Given that epidurals are only available on hospital labour wards, I believe this is a big factor behind why so many people choose hospitals over birth centres and home.

Hopefully by reading this book and learning more, you will begin to feel more confident about your body's ability to birth your baby, and will be able to use your techniques to stay calm and relaxed, so you won't need an epidural. It's worth knowing that gas and air are available at home and in birth centres.

We need to break the fear that surrounds childbirth by changing the stories that we tell, so that people feel less frightened and more confident in choosing a home birth or birth centre, if they'd like to. By being frightened about birth, and starting your labour from a place of anxiety, fear and panic, you're immediately producing adrenaline and making things more complicated than they need to be. It's a bit like a self-fulfilling prophecy! When you fear that birth will be painful and that lots of horrible things will happen, you start birth from a place of fear. You then produce adrenaline, progress is slow and painful, and, as a result, you require pain relief and assistance. The whole experience confirms your belief that birth is horrible, you tell your friend and so the cycle continues.

But it doesn't have to be this way! And I hope that by the time you finish this book you will really believe that it's possible to give birth in a very different and very positive way and to feel hugely empowered by the incredible experience.

Do not underestimate the impact your environment has on how you feel and how your birth pans out. Choose an environment in which you can feel relaxed and comfortable, an environment that is conducive to vaginal birth, if that is what you're hoping for. And when you think about it, home is usually all of those things: safe, familiar, comforting and relaxing. But if home is not a sensible option for you, you are now equipped with the tools to make any space your own oasis of calm.

BIRTH STORY

Positive water birth in hospital – Holly, second-time parent

For all you first-time parents, my first birth was only negative because I felt totally unprepared and had no tools to help guide me through the process, so you are all off to an incredible start in welcoming your baby into the world.

My labour started with irregular surges on Wednesday the 20th. I didn't notice that they were of any significance until around 2pm as I had been experiencing mild period-type cramps on and off for the previous two weeks.

However, after a morning of frantic cleaning while my eldest was at nursery, I sat down for a cuppa and noticed that the mild surges were coming every four to seven minutes, lasting around four seconds. At this point, I felt a bit in denial as my waters broke with my first labour before I had any surges, but this hadn't happened this time round.

Anyway, my husband came home from work and we timed the surges for a while. They continued to come at irregular intervals until about 1am. Up until this point I had put our candles out, used my essential oils and liquid yoga room spray and can honestly say it was a relaxing, if not surreal, experience.

I rang and spoke to the midwives when I felt the time was right and they told me to come in to the hospital. As I expected, the change of location slowed down my surges for a while, but the midwives were very relaxed and very keen for me to dim the lights, get the candles back out and spray my sprays, which was great.

I had a slight wobble and decided I wanted some kind of pain relief (not because I was actually in pain, but I think I felt overwhelmed) as I went into established labour. But my husband was really supportive and talked me back around and the midwife really reminded me to continue with my up breathing (which is amazing for focus).

As the sun came up, the sky looked like it was on fire and was so amazing to see – it made the whole process feel quite magical. I continued with my up breathing and when I was expected to be about 7cm the midwife ran the birthing pool for me.

I spent two hours in the pool, using gas and air for the surges and had lavender on a muslin to smell, which was really relaxing. We also had our playlist on in the background.

When I transitioned into the down stage of labour the sensation and the uncontrollable push from my body were incredible to experience. My midwife was so supportive and didn't want to interfere at all, she just knew from the change in my noises that I was ready to deliver my baby.

I think the difference between my first labour and second labour was the ability to allow my body to do its thing and not fight against a very intense sensation. I can honestly say that I didn't find this experience painful, and actually found it quite nice/satisfying because I was so in awe of what my body was doing. I kept the affirmation that 'my surges are not stronger than me because they are me' firmly in my mind and because of this I feel that I had the best experience of my life so far.

My baby came into the world at 9.46am on the summer solstice in the most incredibly calm way and I am still on the biggest high imaginable. John Lennon's 'Beautiful Boy' was playing as I gave birth, and I know I will never be able to hear this song now without crying.

5

My womb, my rules!

Knowing that you are in charge when it comes to your birth, that any decisions are yours alone to make and that *nothing* can be done to you without your explicit consent should immediately help you to feel more confident, assertive and, most importantly, relaxed. In this chapter I will help you understand your rights so that you feel empowered to ask questions, to seek clarity, to explore options and ultimately take control of your birth, making informed decisions that enable you to welcome your baby into the world in the way you believe is best.

So, let's just get a few things straight. First up, if you're pregnant and reading this book, I'm going to assume you're capable of making your own decisions. Of course, like me, you might be quite indecisive, but all the same, you understand the basic principle that you are an autonomous individual and have the freedom to make your own choices.

Most of us enjoy this freedom and would, quite rightly, stand up for ourselves if we felt this was in any way threatened. And yet, for reasons I can only speculate over, the minute we set foot in a hospital setting, we have a tendency to relinquish all personal responsibility over ourselves, our bodies, our babies and, worryingly, our birth, and hand full responsibility and control over all of the aforementioned into the hands of a doctor or midwife. Why is this?

In a hospital setting, you are *legally* required to give *informed* consent prior to anything being done to you. In reality, on a busy ward, what happens all too often is that someone gives *consent* for a procedure, or an examination, or an intervention, without being fully informed about the path they are now heading down. They just say yes and comply. Often, one thing leads to another – what's known as the cascade of intervention – and the person is left feeling distressed or, worse, traumatised because they didn't understand what was happening or why. They felt out of control and frightened, didn't feel they were part of the decision-making process or even that it was their decision, and had no idea that one thing was likely to lead to the next or that they could say *no*. They therefore come out of the experience feeling shell-shocked, as though it all happened *to* them, rather than that they were an active participant in their own birth experience. This is sadly how many people express feeling about their births.

I have just described what I call 'the conveyor belt of care'. You go through the doors of the hospital (or the birth centre) and are processed through the system with a 'one-size-fits-all' approach. You are periodically assessed and routinely examined for progress as though the expectation is that every parent progresses in the same way, unaffected by external influences or personal circumstances, cervixes dilating like clockwork.

I call it the conveyor belt of *care*, because certainly nobody is trying to cause any harm. I like to trust that everyone involved wishes to provide a good level of care and is committed to the safe delivery of baby, but everyone is also on the clock and overworked in an under-resourced hospital, having to adhere to strict guidelines and without the time to explore other options.

It is the midwives' mantra to provide individualised care, and

I believe midwives, on the whole, passionately want to be able to do just that. It's just that the reality of the situation is quite different, and midwives have so little time and so many people to see. That's why it's so important that *you* (yes, *you* reading this!) step off that conveyor belt – or, better still, avoid getting swept up onto it in the first place – and take control of your birth. I want you to have the confidence to navigate your own birth, in the way that is best for you and your baby, because one size does *not* fit all.

When it comes to giving informed consent, it's a bit of a grey area as to whose responsibility it is to ensure that you are fully informed and therefore in a position to make an informed decision. People might defer to doctors and midwives and other health professionals but, really, the responsibility to ensure you are fully informed is yours. You need to ensure you have all the information you need. That means you're going to have to ask questions! So, never be afraid of asking. Never worry that it's a silly question, that you'll look stupid, are being annoying or wasting anyone's time. Making informed decisions, rather than feeling forced into doing something you don't want or don't understand, is essential to ensuring a positive birth experience, and unfortunately there's no dress rehearsal! So, ask the questions, get the information you need, understand your options and make sure you're in a position to make informed decisions.

Even if you end up agreeing to go with the recommended course of action after asking all your questions (and that's all it ever is: a recommendation), then at least *you* have reached that decision because it feels right for *you* and your baby. Not because you did what you were told. Even though the outcome might seem the same from an outsider's perspective, there is in fact a massive difference. The act of making your own decision is empowering and enables you to embrace your choice feeling positive and in control. The benefits of feeling this way are long-term and profound – a positive experience in birth significantly reduces the risk of suffering from postnatal depression.

So why is it that so many strong, independent, intelligent people cross that threshold into a hospital and forget they can say 'no'? What causes them to forget that it is *their* choice? That they *have* choices!

I believe the reasons are complex but include:

1. We are so conditioned from an early age to respect authority and essentially 'do what we are told', firstly by our parents, then our teachers and, later in life, the law. We live in a society in which we are taught to respect those in a position of authority and comply. This conditioning runs deep and when we feel vulnerable, as we do in labour and birth, we are less able to advocate for ourselves and therefore *more* compliant. We also don't wish to cause a fuss, ruffle any feathers, or be labelled a troublemaker, so, again, we comply, even when we aren't overly happy doing so.

2. We do what we are told because we are often frightened about birth and the unknown and we trust that the medical professionals know more – and better – than us, which in some respects they do, but certainly not all. We also often don't want to go against medical advice because the 'what ifs' plague us, so, again, we defer the decision to others, going with what we are told is best, placing the responsibility for our body, our well-being, our baby and our birth experience in the hands of somebody else. We also often don't feel qualified to challenge the opinion of medical professionals, mistaking our inexperience for inability.

In relation to point 2, it's worth remembering that what is offered by professionals might not necessarily be what is best for you as an individual. Advice given is mediated by a number of factors. For example, within the NHS, what you are offered is a course of action that is deemed safe, but is also time-efficient, cost-efficient and uses the fewest resources. Because, as we all know, the NHS is working to a budget. There are also guidelines that govern NHS practice and, understandably, NHS employees will wish to be compliant and follow those recommended guidelines. Remember, though, that guidelines have been created for the general population, and when it comes to birth a one-size-fits-all approach doesn't always work. The guidelines might not be right for you and your unique situation. Elsewhere in private practice, you might be offered the most expensive option – especially if your insurance is covering the cost! So, for all these reasons, and there are many more, we should never hand complete control over our births to anyone else. Not least because, when it comes to birth, you are the only person in that room who is *feeling* and experiencing the sensations of birth. Nobody else. You are the only person who can explain what is happening inside you and what you are feeling. Only you are able to tap into that powerful instinct. Only you can choose to do what feels right. Only you can make the informed decisions that need to be made. Above all, legally, only you can give consent for anything that is proposed.

3. And then there is the language used by medical professionals, which means recommendations and advice are often delivered sounding like non-negotiable orders. The amount of times I've heard fully grown adults (myself included) being told to 'hop up on the bed' for an examination – with no explanation as to why or what is involved, no

discussion as to whether or not an invasive internal examination is wanted, or whether there are any risks. Just a simple 'hop up on the bed', as though they are a child. It's immediately disempowering and, because of the conditioning that I describe above, the majority of people will go along with it. The medics don't wish to cause harm with the words they use. I suspect it's all said without much conscious consideration and is more down to a lack of being mindful about the impact of language.

Remember, this might be your first birth, your last birth, your only birth – a monumental and life-changing occasion in your life – but for the doctor or midwife looking after you, you could be the third, fourth, fifth, tenth expectant parent they have dealt with today. It might be very routine for them to carry out internal examinations, but, for you, it could be a big deal. So, be mindful of language and always remember: it's a recommendation, never an order. A simple and polite 'Thank you for your advice. I will have a think about what you've suggested and let you know what I decide' works wonders as a reminder to those providing the care that *you* are in charge.

Remember, you have the same human rights in labour as you do in other parts of your life. This includes the right to make your own decisions and choices. That means you can decline anything and everything: it's your right. I'm not advocating that you should, or that it would be sensible, I'm merely reminding you that everything is your choice. And you can *always* say no. You should not feel pressured or coerced into doing something you do not want to do. You have the right for your wishes to be respected. Writing those wishes down makes it even harder to ignore. Handing over a piece of paper with your birth preferences clearly outlined, for example, is a great idea and one that

I highly recommend you do. Essentially it is a written document outlining what you want and don't want to happen in various situations. Medical professionals are obligated to respect your wishes and nothing should ever happen to you without you having given your explicit consent. So, put what's important to you in writing and hand that clear, written statement over to whoever is providing you with care. Have multiple copies with you to account for shift changes.

Above all, remember: it is *your* body, it is *your* baby, it is *your* birth and it is always *your* decision. Remind yourself of this, and the fact that you are in charge!

The more confident you feel going into birth, the more relaxed you will feel. The more relaxed you are, the better your birth will be. So, if there's anything that is causing you to feel anxious, now is the time to quash it! We are out to break that cycle of fear → tension → pain.

Read these facts over and over if necessary and really allow their full meaning to seep in. *You are in charge.* There is no need to worry about things happening *to* you that you do not want to happen, because you can simply say 'no'. You know that now. You have a no in your back pocket and you're free to pull it out whenever you wish. *Everything is your choice.* Allow yourself to feel empowered by this knowledge, and protected by your rights. Remember, remember, remember, you can *always* just say 'no'; you *are* allowed!

6

Use your B.R.A.I.N.

As you now know, your informed consent is required for *every* procedure that takes place in hospital. That means any time an intervention is offered or suggested, no matter how minor or major, it is a legal obligation for you to give your informed consent. Without your consent, anything that happens to you could be considered assault. This makes the issue of 'giving consent' a serious one and an important topic to get to grips with.

Ideally you're now feeling confident and empowered, knowing that you are in charge. That's all well and good, but what happens if things do become challenging and medical professionals are sharing their recommendations? How do you ensure you're not just sitting on that conveyor belt of care? How can you ensure it is *you* who is making the decisions and calling the shots? Most importantly, how can you ensure that you are fully informed and in a position to make those important decisions?

In this chapter I'm going to teach you a very easy but invaluable framework that you can use to ensure you have all the information to make informed decisions. This framework can be used for absolutely everything and it's a good idea to make sure your birth partner is familiar with it as well, as they are more likely to be the one using it when you are in labour.

Remember, not only are you responsible for making the decisions that need to be made, but the responsibility to ensure you're *fully* informed before making any decision is also *yours*. This is important stuff!

So how can you ensure you're making the right choice for you and your baby?

You just need to remember to use your B.R.A.I.N. This handy little framework isn't just useful for navigating birth but, as I said before, it's great for all of life's big decisions. It's another life skill.

So let's run through what B.R.A.I.N. stands for:

B is for BENEFITS
R is for RISKS
A is for ALTERNATIVES
I is for INSTINCT
N is for NOTHING

These are the things you need to establish *before* making any big (or small) decision. By working your way through this list and understanding each element, you're ensuring you have *all* the information available and are in a position to make a properly informed decision that is right for you and your baby.

So let's dig a little deeper.

B is for Benefits

What are the *benefits* of the proposed action/intervention? Essentially these are the 'pros' of accepting and giving consent. If an action or intervention is being offered, it's likely you'll have been told the 'pros' already, but if not, just ask: what are the benefits of saying yes and doing this? Once you've established these, you move on to the next point.

R is for Risks

What are the *risks* of the proposed action/intervention? These are the 'cons' of accepting and giving consent, which you may *not* have been informed about. Essentially, you need to weigh up the pros and cons in order to make a decision. Do the benefits outweigh the risks? Or do you feel the risks are too high?

As much as we'd like to believe that there will always be a straightforward, clear-cut answer here, the likelihood is that most decisions are a little more complex. Occasionally there will be an obvious answer, where the benefits far outweigh any potential risks, but, more often than not, it's a much closer call and people will come to different decisions.

And that, by the way, is totally fine. Your friend, your colleague, your own mum might make a different decision in the same set of circumstances, but what's important is that you go with what's right for *you* and not what someone else would do. Remember, we are all individuals: we have different thresholds for what is acceptable to us, we want different things – or at least different things matter more to different people – and we have all had different life experiences. We are not going to always make the same choices. That's the beauty of being an autonomous individual.

This nugget of advice extends well into parenting and all the debates that you will have to navigate: breast vs bottle, co-sleeping vs a standalone crib, baby-led weaning vs purees. Being a parent means facing a never-ending series of seemingly serious and important decisions that need to be made, decisions about which everyone has a strong opinion. But the only opinion that ever matters is yours. Remember: *your* body, *your* baby, *your* choice! Learning to not be influenced by others, but rather feeling sure of your own decisions, trusting you know best for your baby is another life skill.

So, ask explicitly what the risks are of saying yes and consenting to what's being offered. There are *always* potential risks or 'cons' when making decisions. Nothing is so straightforward in life that it can be guaranteed to be 100 per cent safe and without *any* chance of negative implications. Life isn't so black and white. Understand what the potential negative consequences could be, and weigh this up against the benefits to decide what course of action feels best for you.

A is for Alternatives

What are the *alternatives* to the proposed action/intervention? This is an important one to ask and consider within the pros vs cons mix. Are there any alternatives? Often there are. And it might well be the case that these are preferable to you.

As I said before, what's usually offered by the NHS is a course of action that is considered safe, first and foremost, but one that is also *cost-effective*. This means there are often alternatives that are not offered up as the first option, because perhaps they cost more, take longer or use more resources.

A good example of this is induction. The NICE guidelines state that you should be offered increased antenatal monitoring at least twice weekly as an alternative to induction. This is rarely offered in practice and, unless you know about this or think to ask about alternatives, you won't even know this is an option available to you. This means you might potentially agree to an induction without understanding its associated risks, and without knowing you had any other options – that there were alternatives. I've heard this so many times and, indeed, lived this experience with my first.

So always ask, are there any alternatives? Sometimes when it comes to things progressing slowly, you might be offered an intervention to speed things up. However, if baby is well and you are well, you might well decide that a good alternative course of action would be to dim the lights, remove unnecessary people from the room, do a little relaxation practice and get your natural oxytocin flowing again.

There's a great quote I always mention at this point when teaching and that's:

'If I don't know my options, I don't have any' (Diane Korte).

Do not be afraid to ask and establish what your options are. There are always options and it's always your choice.

I is for Instinct

What is your *instinct* telling you? Your instinct is a powerful thing and is part of the reason we are all still here today! All mammals behave instinctively and although we have, of course, evolved, we are still mammals with this powerful intuition within us. The problem is we tend to forget and ignore our instincts because we have been conditioned to process everything and make decisions with our heads rather than our instincts!

In birth, when you are deep in the zone, your instinct will be even more powerful than it has ever been before. It will take over. It will be almost tangible. You will feel your body do amazing things and know what is happening within. Midwives should encourage you to listen to your body and do what it needs to do. Nothing is more powerful than your own instinct in birth. It's highly tuned. So tap into it and don't be afraid to do so.

Remember, you may be surrounded by experienced birth professionals with years of experience working on a labour ward, you may be a first-time parent, you may never have done this before, but you are the only person in the room who can *feel* what is happening! You can feel reassured and confident knowing that you *do* know what's happening and you *do* know what's best, because it's happening inside you! You know your body better than anyone else, it's your body after all. You will know what feels comfortable and right for you, and what doesn't. Don't be afraid to let your instinct guide you.

When it comes to making decisions, when you weigh up the pros and cons, when you consider the alternatives, remember also to listen to your instinct – what feels like the right course of action for *you*. You know you! What does your gut tell you to do?

Parental instinct is established in pregnancy and certainly it's very active in birth. You know best. Listen to that powerful instinct of yours. Take it into consideration. Ask yourself: does this course of action or proposed intervention *feel* right for me and my baby?

N is for Nothing

What happens if we do *nothing*?

This final question always seems like a bit of a throwaway one – an afterthought. But actually, it can sometimes be the most important one to ask.

What happens if we do nothing ... for five minutes? Ten minutes? An hour? Four hours? Twenty-four hours? A few days? Another week?

You see where I'm going with this ... Depending on the situation you find yourself in, the timescales might shift. If things seem critical you might be asking for a few minutes to get yourself into the right head space; if your waters have broken and you're feeling under pressure to agree to an induction because labour has not yet started spontaneously, you might be asking for a few hours; if your baby is breech and you're considering a planned caesarean you might be asking for a few more days to make your decision and to give your baby the opportunity to turn; or if there are concerns about baby's growth (big or small) you might ask to review the situation in a week and opt for monitoring in the interim.

There are too many potential scenarios for me to list here, but asking for a bit of time when making a decision (even just a couple of minutes) is almost always a good idea. I say 'almost' because we know that emergencies can happen, as they can in any area of life or any given day. And in the extremely rare event that a true emergency is unfolding, it might not be appropriate to delay. A true emergency, in which every minute matters, is the only situation where asking for some time might not be helpful. In *all* other situations, asking for time is hugely beneficial. If you feel you're being put under pressure or rushed and you've established it's *not* a medical emergency then you can *always* ask for some time – even if it is just a few minutes. In that time you can process the new information, ask any necessary questions, reach the right decision for you and your baby, and be in a position to give *informed* consent.

In the majority of cases, being rushed into making a decision or put under pressure results in more negative than positive feelings long-term, leaving room for regret and what ifs. Nobody likes feeling that they were forced into something. We enjoy and value our own free will! Reaching a decision *yourself*, even if it means opting for whatever was initially proposed, will leave you feeling empowered and confident as you navigate your birth and any twists, turns and deviations from the initial 'plan' it might take. These feelings around your birth will stick with you forever, so make sure they are happy positive ones. Don't be rushed into anything or pressured to conform to a one-size-fits-all approach.

If there's ever any doubt as to whether or not the situation is an emergency one, simply ask the question: Is this a medical emergency? You should be able to trust that the team providing your care will be honest, and if they confirm it's an emergency, then stand back and allow them to do their lifesaving work. In real emergency situations it's normal for the person giving birth to be put to sleep under a general anaesthetic and for the birth partner to be asked to leave the room. However, real emergencies are *extremely* rare. And if we got caught up worrying about every tiny risk that exists in life, then we might never leave the house. Life-threatening emergencies can, quite literally, happen anywhere – crossing the road, for example. But thankfully they are rare and extremely so when it comes to giving birth.

The *process* of making the decision and using your B.R.A.I.N. is an important one to work through and is what offers long-term benefits from a mental health perspective. Often, we get so caught up in 'the plan' or focused on this single image of what our dream birth should look like that we start to believe any deviation from 'the plan' is a failing and means we didn't get the birth we wanted. I encourage you to think differently... it's not what birth *looks* like that matters – ultimately it doesn't really matter if you're at home, or in a pool or in theatre – what really matters most is how you *felt* during that experience. It's the *feelings* attached to the memories that last a lifetime and not the mechanics of how a baby entered the world. You might well have created a set of preferences (and it's definitely a good idea to do so) but they need to be adaptable: pregnancy and birth can be unpredictable. A positive birth, which is something we all strive for, is a birth experience that leaves you feeling empowered rather than traumatised, where your wishes are respected, you're listened to and feel calm, confident and informed. Water birth, caesarean birth, whatever – it's not a particular *type* of birth.

Having helped many thousands of people prepare to give birth and seen them come out the other side, I know this to be true: it's perfectly possible to have a positive experience wherever and however you give birth. You may have a dreamy water birth at home, you may have a planned gentle caesarean or even an unplanned caesarean, but all of these births can be positive, empowering and happy experiences. On the flipside, having spoken to so many people about their previous birth experiences, I know that it's equally possible to suffer from postnatal depression and post-traumatic stress disorder after an unplanned caesarean as it is after a birth that might appear straightforward and uncomplicated on paper. Just because someone had a vaginal birth in water without pain relief, it doesn't mean it felt like a positive experience for them. They may have felt frightened, panicked, unsupported; they may not have felt respected or listened to, and they might not have understood what was happening. These are the things that can make birth feel traumatic.

So, can we make sure we have a positive experience whilst remaining open-minded as to how that birth happens? Can *all* births really be positive? The answer is *yes*! If someone feels in control as they navigate their birth experience, feels calm, confident and well supported and is empowered to be able to make the best decisions for themself and their baby then, even if 'the plan' changes, they can still feel that it was a positive experience because they know in their heart that they brought their baby into the world in the best way possible on that day. And that is what matters. So, take your time to make the decisions that need to be made. Ask that vital question; what happens if we do nothing for x amount of time?

Let's try out the B.R.A.I.N. method using internal examinations as an example. They might be routinely conducted, but . . .

- They're invasive
- They can be uncomfortable
- They can hinder your relaxation and make you feel anxious
- They can cause the cervix to regress and close up
- They don't give you any indication of how long there is left to go
- They don't let you know anything about baby's well-being
- The measurement is subjective
- There's a risk of rupturing the membranes
- And a risk of introducing infection

If you apply the B.R.A.I.N. framework and weigh up the benefits (knowing approximately how many centimetres dilated you are and whether you're making measurable progress) against the risks (outlined above) you might decide the risks outweigh the benefits. Or, you may feel the benefits outweigh the risks. You might choose to decline *all* examinations or just some. You could always opt to defer the initial examination, usually offered on arrival at a birth centre or hospital, until the point at which you feel settled into the new space and relaxed. It's absolutely your choice as to when or even *if* you have an internal examination.

Remember, too, the 'A' from your B.R.A.I.N. framework. A is for Alternatives and there are other ways to assess progress. These include using a mirror so that the midwife can *see* what is happening without having to invasively examine you or even touch or disturb you. Also, through observation: are the surges coming more frequently, are they lasting longer, are they becoming stronger? What sounds are being made? All of these things are indicators that labour is progressing well.

Don't forget to tap into your instinct. Will this examination *aid* your relaxation? Will it tell you anything important? Remember, internal examinations aren't normally used to check on baby's well-being; baby's well-being is monitored by listening in regularly to their heartbeat. And an internal examination can never tell you how long is left! Which is what most parents want to know. You can dilate very quickly or slow down depending on so many factors – many of them external and environmental factors. So, knowing how dilated you are in this moment doesn't indicate how long it will be until you are fully dilated. Also, it's an *estimate* with someone's fingers, and that someone may as well be blindfolded. It's not exact.

And then, N for Nothing! Ask if there are any potential negative consequences to declining an internal examination at this time. You can *always* decline or postpone an internal examination. It is your choice. You have the absolute right.

Mind-blowing game-changer fact

Nobody has the right to put their fingers inside your vagina without your consent, or pressure you into saying yes. Not in a nightclub (where it would be considered sexual assault) and not in a hospital. It may seem obvious but so many people have told me they thought they *had* to have internal examinations.

No matter how seemingly innocuous or routine what's being suggested appears to be, always engage your B.R.A.I.N. prior to making any decision, and, more crucially, before saying yes and giving consent. Do not be afraid to ask questions! It is your responsibility to ensure you are fully informed and the easiest and best way of getting informed is to ask questions of the experts. Never feel you're being difficult by doing so, or that you're not equipped to challenge medical professionals. I'll say it time and time again: this is *your* body, *your* baby, *your* birth and most importantly *your* choice! You're in charge! And just in case you're having a wobble in confidence, always remember you are a strong, capable individual and well able to make the right decisions for yourself and your baby. You're growing a human. You're a walking miracle! And a bloody *superhero*! Never forget it.

Finally, make sure your birth partner(s) are familiar with this B.R.A.I.N. framework too, because when you're in active labour you might not be in a position to think clearly, ask questions, process the information and advocate for yourself. If you're in the zone and breathing deeply through your surges, you're going to need your birth partner to step up here and help you by gathering the information on your behalf. So, make sure they know to ask: What are the benefits? What are the risks? Are there any alternatives? What happens if we do nothing for the next ten minutes? They can then relay this information to you between surges and you can weigh up the pros and cons, consider the alternatives and check in with your powerful instinct to make the decision that's right for you and your baby. Your birth partner cannot make any decision for you – you need to be the one to give informed consent – but they can help massively by stepping up, using their B.R.A.I.N. and asking the necessary questions. You can imagine how easy it would be otherwise – when in the midst of labour – to get swept along that conveyor belt of care, consenting to things without fully understanding the whole picture. When you are in active, established labour you are vulnerable, and this is when you need your birth partner most to advocate for you, ensure your wishes are respected and get the facts for you if new decisions need to be made.

Fold the corner down on this chapter and get your birth partner(s) to read it. I mean, ideally, they'll read this whole book, but if that's not looking likely, get them to at least read this bit!

BIRTH STORY

Positive hospital birth – Hayley, second-time parent

My baby was born about two hours after arriving at the delivery suite after my surges started naturally at forty-one weeks and one day. It was a vaginal birth with no pain relief and very little interference from the midwives (one student and one midwife), with en caul and weighing 7lb 2oz. My baby is absolutely perfect!

The midwives were so incredibly supportive and respectful of our wishes. I could feel early on that baby was back to back (as was my first baby), but they only told me after the birth so as not to be in any way discouraging. They barely spoke, only offering encouragement towards the end of a surge. I must say my husband was an incredible support, and, together with the midwives, I felt so safe that I was able to keep my eyes closed and focus on listening to my music.

The biggest difference between this and my first baby's birth was my taking control of my care throughout rather than relying on people to tell me what was going to happen. I'm not the most confident of people but the feeling of empowerment that Siobhan instilled in me is remarkable. I was able to communicate with my husband about the birth so he understood the importance of being calm and quiet and in control. I was able to communicate better and confide in my community midwives, who were all very interested in hypnobirthing (if not entirely experienced) and supportive, and I had the confidence to question the consultant (who was very kind but still from a very medical place, of course) and after using my B.R.A.I.N. avoided later growth scans which were causing unnecessary stress to me and my husband.

I'm so incredibly grateful. I feel confident and relaxed with my new baby and I'm thrilled to be home with my family. Hypno-birthing really has been a game changer. And babies really do come when they're ready!'

7

Keeper of the cave: the role of the birth partner

The keeper of the cave is the phrase I use to describe the role of the birth partner. Back in prehistoric times you can imagine people would have typically given birth in the safety of a cave (or some other private space). Someone would have been appointed to mind the entrance and keep guard. This person would have been responsible for physically protecting the sacred birthing space from potential predators or attack. When giving birth you are vulnerable in the sense that you are not able to defend yourself. The same goes for newborn babies!

You actually still see this happening in the wild today: when an animal is giving birth, often another member of the group can be seen protecting the space and keeping guard.

Nowadays, hopefully, you're not giving birth in a cave! You're a lot more likely to be in a birth centre or hospital, if not at home. Of course the space no longer needs protection from savage animals and there should be no threat of attack. However, the role of the birth partner – the keeper of the cave – has certainly not become redundant. The role has evolved: the environment may have changed but the need to protect the space in order to maintain a sense of peace and calm, enabling the body to soften and open and for birth to happen, is just as important as it ever was.

Birth partners play an essential role in labour and birth and need to a) be recognised for the important part they play and b) understand themselves how important their presence and involvement are. A good birth partner can make the world of difference when it comes to birth.

Depending on your situation, your birth partner could be your partner, your parent, another family member, a friend or a doula. It doesn't really matter *who* the birth partner is as long as they make you feel safe, they understand your wishes and you trust them to advocate for you if necessary. Knowing that you have a birth partner you trust – by your side to support you, and on your side to advocate for you – enables you to let go of what is going on around you, channel your focus and really relax deeply into the experience.

When it comes to protecting the space these days, it's less about *physically* defending the person giving birth from attack, and more about shielding them from interruptions, which can be frequent, especially in a busy hospital setting. These interruptions, however routine or mundane, can negatively impact the progression of labour. The more frequent the interruptions, the more significant the overall impact. Interruptions do not aid relaxation and therefore need to be kept to a minimum. At worst, frequent interruptions from strangers can cause labour to slow or even stall as it triggers the production of adrenaline, which we know results in the surges becoming less efficient, labour becoming longer, little progress being made and also for everything to feel more uncomfortable. This can easily cause someone to enter the negative cycle of fear → tension → pain, which is to be avoided at all costs!

A simple way to protect the space from unwelcome interruptions is to have a copy of the birth preferences clearly outlined in writing, and to ensure that everyone providing care also has a copy and has been requested to read the document. Hopefully, this will be enough to ensure that the wishes of the person giving birth are respected, but if not, birth partners will need to step up and advocate at this point. This is the modern-day version of protecting the space from attack. You do not need to be directly confrontational. I appreciate this doesn't come easily to everyone and, in any case, will probably be unnecessary, but it's possible to be polite whilst insisting that the birth preferences are read and respected. Remind those present why you want the space to be calm and quiet, and how you are working to help the person giving birth achieve a state of deep relaxation. Let those who are providing the care know that you've been learning about hypnobirthing and practising the techniques. I've no doubt that, in the vast majority of cases, you will encounter midwives who will go above and beyond to support and accommodate everyone's wishes and you will have no issues whatsoever. But, in the unlikely event that you do face opposition, be prepared to speak up and protect the space – metaphorical spear in hand!

Think back for a moment to the 'perfect' environment for vaginal birth – the environment that animals instinctively choose. It's a dark, quiet and private one. Hospitals tend to be the exact opposite: brightly lit, noisy, busy and full of strangers. Now you may well be choosing to birth in a different setting to avoid just that, and that's great, but if you are opting for hospital or indeed transferring into hospital for whatever reason, you need to be prepared to transform the room, making it as close as possible to that dark, quiet, private space that is optimal for birth. You have your five senses checklist to help you with this and a well-packed birth bag full of everything you need to make this happen.

Use the traffic light system

I devised this 'traffic light' system idea a while ago to help birth partners understand what their role might look like on a surge-by-surge basis and I think it's pretty useful (if I do say so myself!).
So here goes ...

Green The green state is the optimum state and the one we are all aiming for in which the parent is completely relaxed and at ease. If I refer to 'the green state' or 'returning to green', this is what I mean: returning to a state of deep relaxation in mind and body, not feeling anxious about anything, with no tension anywhere in the body.

Through practice you will become very familiar with what this lovely green state feels like and will be able to easily switch off to access this state more and more quickly over time.

Red The red state is the one we want to avoid at all costs. This is where someone is panicking and producing lots of adrenaline. This causes the blood (and oxygen) to be redirected to their limbs and away from their uterus muscles. Very quickly the surges will become less efficient and increasingly uncomfortable, lengthening the labour. If someone appears to hit the red, that's when the birth partner needs to use all of the tools in their toolkit – and quickly!

Amber As you've probably guessed, amber is the in-between state. There is some anxiety, some muscle tension. Amber is a spectrum. It's normal to teeter into amber during a powerful surge. However, if you edge further and further into amber with each surge, you run the risk of hitting red. Therefore, it's the birth partner's job to look out for signs that could indicate that someone is in amber (tense shoulders, tense jaw, tight grip, voicing worries) and use the appropriate tool from the toolkit to help them return to the green state.

For example, if the birth partner notices that the shoulders of the person giving birth are creeping up towards their ears, they might rest their hands on their shoulders and remind them to relax. If they notice that they are gripping something tightly, they might use the arm-stroking technique. If their jaw is tense, they might use an arm drop to encourage them to release and let go. If they are voicing worries and doubting themself, then some reassuring words or positive affirmations might be needed. The birth partner can use any of the tools at their disposal to help the person in labour return to the happy green state.

If you were to plot someone's progress through the surges on a special traffic-light-themed graph, what we'd probably see is that each time a surge builds and peaks, the person teeters towards amber and then, as the surge releases, they relax back into green. The birth partner is there to support and coach the person giving birth through each surge and, once the surge has passed, can use techniques to speed up this return to green. Moving between green and the bottom of amber is fine, and to be expected. What we want to avoid is moving towards red and having no tools to bring us back to the green.

So, birth partners, use the counting during the surge (if that's what is wanted) and then the other relaxation tools between the surges in the few minutes of rest time. Pause what you are doing when the next surge comes on and return to the counting, then, once it has passed, you can resume whatever it was you were doing: arm stroking, light-touch massage, relaxation reading, etc.

And if you're giving birth, remember: it's all about the green state of absolute relaxation.

I really can't emphasise enough the importance of the birth partner's role, and the difference an attentive, supportive, informed and empowered birth partner can make to a person's birth experience. It's easy to dismiss the role of the birth partner as insignificant, because, just as people are generally conditioned to believe that birth is dramatic and traumatic, we are equally conditioned to believe that birth partners are useless! Think of every movie you've ever seen in which birth has been depicted: birth partners are shown to be annoying and unhelpful, and even a complete liability and the butt of all jokes.

Just as I encourage those who are pregnant to actively build new, *positive* associations with birth through watching positive birth videos, reading positive birth stories, listening to positive affirmations and absorbing positive imagery from birth photography, it's also important that birth partners do the same. Birth partners will benefit from watching these videos and reading these stories because they will get a better idea of what their role *really* looks like. Without this, the only template they probably have is what they have seen on TV growing up. And that's certainly not the image we want birth partners to base their expectations on.

Hypnobirthing, as an approach to birth, seeks to involve the birth partner as much as possible. It really is just as much for the birth partner's benefit as it is for the person giving birth: an empowered birth partner goes into birth feeling informed and confident and is able to actively (and practically) support someone through the labour, whilst enabling them to navigate any twists and turns in the best way possible. By doing so, birth partners come out the other side feeling a huge sense of achievement, one of empowerment, because they played such a big part in something so momentous. This, sadly, is not how all birth partners feel post-birth. Many can feel quite traumatised themselves by the birth, looking on and not knowing how to help. They report feeling powerless, unable to help the person they love, scared about what's happening and left in the dark throughout the experience. And, worst of all, afterwards they feel they cannot 'complain' or even share their feelings because the focus is, naturally, on the experience of the person who has just given birth, so they tend to suffer in silence. Hypnobirthing aims to help birth partners feel involved, to understand what is going on, to have a clear job and a to-do list to work through. Most birth partners I've taught over the years have found having a clearly defined list of practical things they can do to be hugely helpful as they navigate the unknown.

Finally, we have talked about how birth partners need to be an advocate and ensure the birth preferences are respected and how they need to take charge of maintaining a calm, tranquil and dimly lit environment, but aside from all of that, which falls under the gatekeeper/keeper of the cave analogy, birth partners also have the job of supporting the person giving birth through each and every surge using their toolkit. This is why sometimes it can be helpful to have more than one birth partner. Each time the person in labour experiences a surge, birth partners, it falls under your remit to count for them, offer words of reassurance and coach them through, offer drinks and snacks when appropriate, encourage them into good U.F.O. positions and help them return to the green state between surges using either light-touch massage, positive affirmations, arm stroking, the arm-drop technique or your guided relaxation exercises. Birth partners are no longer relegated to the corner of the room to act as an onlooker but play a crucial, hands-on role in the birth.

It's probably worth mentioning that it's totally normal to feel overwhelmed or nervous about what lies ahead, especially if you're being a birth partner for the first time – it's that common fear of the unknown, coupled with all the negative imagery and stories we have been fed our whole lives. But know that, firstly, you're on the cusp of something truly incredible. Couples who have done hypnobirthing together regularly report feeling that the birth experience was a *shared* experience, that they felt like a *team* and that they worked *together* to bring their baby into the world. Many report feeling very close and connected to one another throughout the experience, and as they share the magical and miraculous moment of birth. It *really* can be wonderful, although I appreciate this is not what you normally see on TV. Secondly, know that just by being *present* in the space, even if you do nothing else, you are offering reassurance. You are the familiar person, the trusted and chosen birth partner, in what can be an unfamiliar environment. You are the anchor. You are the keeper of the cave.

BIRTH STORY

Home birth of first-time mum Katie – from the perspective of her birth partner, the baby's father, Jonathan

I arrived home at about 9.20am to find Katie in the bath. We looked at each other and knew this was it. We both cried at this point as we knew we would be meeting our baby soon. We sat and chatted for a bit about what was going on, then started to time the contractions as they were pretty frequent and getting more intense. 'I don't think it will be long – you better get the pool ready' was her instruction. So I dutifully scurried off and got cracking. I got the pool inflated and turned our living room into the nest. I drew the curtains, put the music on, sprayed the room and watched the water trickle into the pool. Honestly, it felt like I could have filled it quicker with a mug! They say a watched kettle never boils. I can now add 'a watched birth pool never fills' to this.

I had called the triage before I started getting the room ready and they said the on-call midwife would ring. Katie came down and was now really working hard with her surges. She was focused and in the zone. Since the pool was still not ready for her she just leant over the birth ball. I kept her hydrated, offered light-touch massage and tried to be positive but calm. It was at this point that the midwife called. She was on another call and would be about half an hour.

The pool was finally ready, Katie got in and you could see the change in her – she just totally relaxed and 'sank' into the warm water. I think it was about now that I 'lost' her, she was totally in the zone, it was quite awesome to watch: she was just breathing through the surges. Our midwife arrived at this point and I felt a bit of relief that I was not on my own any more.

The next bit is all a bit of a blur really. We had regular heart-beat checks and things progressed really well. The odd time she struggled to find a beat, but I knew not to panic as sometimes they are hard to find. Things started to get a bit closer now and the midwife was checking Katie from behind. Katie entered the down phase about now. She had the fight-or-flight transition moment we spoke about on her course and I knew it was my job to calm her down. She was looking a bit hot so I grabbed some ice and just stroked it up and down her arms, whilst telling her how amazingly she was doing – that she was so close. I went down the 'business end' just as Katie had a massive surge and was lucky enough to see my son's head crown. This was an incredible moment and one I will always remember. I rushed back to Katie, held her arms and said: 'One more push, babe, and we get to meet our baby!' And lo and behold, one more push and he was here. Our baby had entered the world!

Katie was incredible. She hardly whimpered through it all, had zero pain relief and we had a super-quick birth – just four hours or so. My advice for expectant parents is to listen to your instincts, dig in and prepare to be amazed.

8

It's as easy as 1, 2, 3

Now that you understand how your body works in labour, you're hopefully feeling confident and empowered, equipped with a set of tools you can use to make your birth the positive experience you want. You're *almost* ready for action!

We've talked about the 'up stage' of labour, in which the cervix dilates and opens, and the 'down stage' of labour, where the baby descends and is born, but now I'm going to tell you that there is a *little* more to it than that.

There are in fact three stages of labour (four, actually, if you include early labour) and although very different things happen in every stage, each is as significant and important as the rest. You'll notice, however, that there are many more than three (or four) terms used to describe the different stages of labour and it can be confusing to say the least! So, in order to make things clear, in this chapter I'm going to break it all down, so you understand what is happening at each stage, from start to finish, and when to use the hypnobirthing techniques you've learnt.

In hospitals, and indeed within your birth notes, the stages of labour are identified in chronological order simply as 'first', 'second' and 'third' stage. Midwives will generally document in your notes how long each stage lasts.

You are said to have entered the 'first stage' of labour once you are 4cm dilated. This means that upon an internal examination (*not* mandatory), your cervix is deemed to be approximately 4cm open. This first stage ends when you're believed to be fully dilated, i.e. when your cervix has opened to approximately 10cm. This stage is also referred to as 'established labour' or 'active labour', and in hypnobirthing this is what we call the 'up stage' – where the muscles of the uterus are drawing *up*, you are doing your *up* breathing through each surge, and your cervix is softening and opening.

You may have spotted a few flaws in the descriptions here already.

Firstly, if the 'first' stage *begins* when you are already 4cm dilated... what goes before? Is there a *pre*-first stage? Well, that's why I mentioned that there are actually *four* stages. *Everything* that happens before being 4cm dilated is counted as 'early labour' or 'the latent phase'. For some, early labour will be less than an hour as things quickly become established, but for others early labour can be days with on-and-off, irregular surges.

Luckily, things tend to progress a little more predictably once labour is well established.

The second flaw you might have spotted is that there is a lot of talk about measurements: the first stage is timed from when you are 4cm dilated through to 10cm. So how do you know when the first stage has begun? How do you know if things are established? How do you even measure the cervix?

In answer to the last hypothetical question, to 'measure' how many centimetres you are dilated requires you to have an internal examination. A midwife or doctor will place their index and middle fingers inside your vagina, reach upwards and just into the cervix and then spread their two fingers apart and estimate (guess) how many centimetres open the gap is. It's not an exact measurement by any stretch (excuse the pun) of the imagination.

It's just an approximate estimate. And obviously when you're at home in early labour you will have no idea how many centimetres open your cervix is – and I'm certainly not encouraging you to try and find out for yourself! In place of internal examinations and measurements, you can gauge (less invasively) how things are progressing by timing the *frequency* of the surges, their *duration* and noting their *intensity*. This is something I'd encourage you to do when at home in early labour and, you'll be happy to know, there is now an app to help you with that! You'll find it listed in the resources section at the back of this book.

Once your surges have started coming they will, at some point, build in all three ways: frequency, duration and intensity. For some people, the surges might become more frequent at first, but last only twenty seconds or so. Others will get nice, strong surges that last a good minute but remain irregular. Labour begins differently for everyone, and even for the same person from one birth to the next: no two are ever the same. So, (admittedly) somewhat unhelpfully, there are no rules. But what you *can* rely on is that, at some point, all three elements will come together and you will be having three surges in every ten-minute period (frequency), each surge will last approximately forty-five seconds to one minute (duration) and they will be good and strong (intensity). It's at *this* point that you can consider yourself to be in established labour (without measurement) and *this* would be the time to travel into the birth centre or hospital, or to call your midwife out to you if having a home birth. (You will usually be advised of the protocol in your area at your thirty-four-week midwife appointment when discussing your birthplace choice.)

This is also known as the magic 3/10/45 and is worth remembering so as to save yourself unnecessary trips to and from the birth centre or hospital: you will usually be sent home if you travel in too soon and things are not yet established/you're not yet 4cm dilated. So remember: you want a regular pattern of three surges every ten minutes, with each surge lasting at least forty-five seconds.

The first stage of labour (up stage)

In hypnobirthing we refer to this first stage of established labour as the 'up stage', as I discussed in the chapter on breathing. We call it the *up* stage because the uterus muscles are drawing *up*, and every time you experience a surge you will feel the muscles tighten and lift, like a wave, to a peak of intensity, and then release. The feeling is really a lot like waves. Whilst this is happening, and the outer layer of the uterus muscles draws up with each surge, the cervix is softening, shortening and then opening.

This is when you use your up breathing: close your eyes, inhale through your nose, for a count of four, feel your chest rise and expand and think to yourself 'inhale peace'. Then, exhale slowly through your mouth for a count of eight, feeling all your muscles relax and release, thinking to yourself 'exhale tension'. Repeat this four times whilst experiencing a surge and then, once you've completed the four repetitions, the surge will have passed and you can go back to your regular breathing. Every time you feel another surge come, you do the same again: in for four, out for eight, four times over. And that's it! Up breathing for the up stage of labour.

This first stage/up stage/established or active labour stage – the real deal if you will – is usually the longest stage of labour. The second stage, also known as the down stage (where you birth your baby), is normally significantly shorter. The up stage is likely to be several hours, whereas the down stage can be anything from a few minutes through to a maximum of around two hours.

The good news is that throughout the up stage you'll be using your up-breathing technique, which is a lovely, calming, relaxing breath and feels nice to do. You'll also be enjoying the light-touch massage, the arm stroking and of course being waited on with drinks and treats. You'll ideally be soaking up the full spa-like experience with room spray, candle lights and spa music playing. It may be several hours, but it can be several glorious hours where you feel fantastic!

Transition

Once you're fully dilated, you may be aware of a transition. Transition simply means transitioning from one stage of labour to the next. In this case the first stage to the second stage – the up stage to the down stage. However, transition can be experienced in different ways.

For some people, transition is seamless and goes unnoticed – one minute they're having a regular surge and the next minute their body is pushing involuntarily and they know they have entered the down stage of labour. For others there is a noticeable change – the surges slow down and become more gentle, almost as if their body is giving them an opportunity to rest before the next stage. Some people have a 'wobble', or slight panic. It's thought the reason for this is that the body releases a small amount of adrenaline so that the senses are heightened, which provides the opportunity to check the environment one last time to make sure it's safe, before the baby makes its descent and is born.

It's common at this point for people to doubt themselves and say they can't do it, or that they want be somewhere else or they want an epidural. The good news is that this moment of panic passes quickly, which is why so many people refer to it as 'a wobble'. The key thing is that birth partners remain calm and offer reassurance, reminding the person in labour that they have done all the hard work now and are so close to meeting their baby.

The second stage of labour (down stage)

Now on to the 'second stage', as it will state in your maternity notes, or the 'down stage' as we call it in hypnobirthing. This is the stage in which baby descends down the birth canal and is born.

The second stage, or the 'down stage', is likely to be much shorter than the first stage. You have already done most of the hard work by dilating to 10cm, so it's now 'just' a case of baby moving down a few inches and being born. Lots of people seem to worry about this stage more than any others. I think there is a tendency to fixate on the *moment* of birth and the effort it will take – not helped of course by every depiction of a baby being born in the media ever! But actually, the majority of the 'hard' work will already have been done. And this moment, the one where your baby actually passes through and is born into the world is relatively quick in comparison and can feel amazing! You will feel your body work powerfully and you get to *feel* your baby for the first time as they move down and are born. It can be utterly incredible and something parents want to do over and over again. Really!

The most helpful thing you can do at this stage is to *relax*. Allow *everything* to soften and open and stretch as it's designed to. The more relaxed you are, the easier and quicker this stage will be, for you and your baby. Gravity also helps massively. In contrast, if you are fearful, everything will tense up and you will effectively slow down the descent of your baby and make it more difficult for your baby to be born without assistance. So, try and reframe so that you look forward to this stage and meeting your baby. When you feel your body begin to push downwards and you feel baby descend, you know you are now *so* close to holding your baby in your arms! I get goosebumps just thinking about it. It is the most amazing sensation.

As we've already discussed, this is called the down stage because the muscles of the uterus change direction now and the inner layer of the uterus muscles begins to push down powerfully with each surge. The baby moves down the birth canal and is born. To keep things simple and straightforward and easy to remember, during the down stage of labour you do your down breathing: take a nice, quick breath in through the nose, feel your lungs expand and then exhale through the mouth, but with focus and intent. Channel your exhalation down through your body and feel your muscles move downwards with your breath. You want to ensure you're working *with* your body and not against it!

This stage is also sometimes referred to as the 'pushing stage'. If you've ever seen someone give birth in a film, as we have already discussed, they are always lying on their backs, legs often in stirrups, red in the face, sweaty and swearing whilst being coached aggressively to push. This is at best an oft-repeated, boring Hollywood narrative and at worst, harmful and destructive – an example of how the media is responsible for conditioning us to believe that birth is something to fear. The good news is that this is categorically *not* how birth should be or, indeed, how it actually is in real life. It's very common to believe that in this down stage of labour you need to actively push or force your baby out with great effort. I believe this is mainly because it's all we've ever seen happen when birth is shown on TV. This, however, is not true.

Your *body* will push your baby out! Your uterus muscles – specifically the inner layer of horizontal rings that have been gathered upwards during the up stage of labour, and which are now bunched in a thick band at the top of your uterus – will, in the down stage of labour, begin to push downwards powerfully with each surge. It's these muscles that will push your baby out. *You* don't need to actively push. You just need to relax and allow your body to do what it's designed to do. Trust your body! Your uterus is a finely tuned muscle that has evolved perfectly over millions of years. Trust your uterus! It knows what to do.

People always tend to stare in disbelief upon hearing this because it's at such odds with their expectations. But it's true. If you were unconscious (hopefully that will never be the case) your body would still be capable of birthing your baby! Those muscles are powerful and perfectly designed. It's not that no pushing needs to take place – something needs to push! Your baby won't just plop out. But it's your body, your muscles which will do the pushing. You don't need to actively force or push anything.

One of the reasons why this stage can sometimes take a long time is that the person giving birth will, without realising, be bracing and drawing up their pelvic floor and tensing all their core muscles. This creates an internal struggle or battle between the muscle groups: the uterus muscles working hard to try and birth the baby and the other muscles tensing, tightening and drawing up to prevent the descent of the baby. That's why the best thing you can do is relax and breathe through the surges and by doing so, allow your uterus muscles to work to their full potential and birth your baby quickly, easily and gently.

Mind-blowing game-changer fact

You do not need to forcibly *push* to get your baby out! Your body is designed to do the job. Just go with your body and avoid tensing and hindering progress. Use your breath to help your muscles do their job. Work *with* your body, not against it.

The only reason you would possibly be advised to push or have a midwife or doctor coaching you to push – which is called *coached* pushing – is if the baby is in distress and therefore there is a need to speed up the birth, or because you're on your back and therefore haven't got gravity on your side and, as a consequence, might need to put some extra effort in because your uterus muscles, powerful as they are, might not be able to push a baby uphill and out! If you've had an epidural this could be the reason why you're on your back on the bed and would increase the need for coached pushing, partly because your body hasn't got gravity on its side, but also because you can't feel when your body is surging/pushing so a midwife would let you know and coach you to push during each surge.

But if all is well, and you're in a good, upright, forward and open position, then there is no need to speed up birth and you can trust that your body will do its job. Trust that uterus!

The time of the second stage or down stage of labour is recorded in your notes as being the time it takes from when you're fully dilated through to the birth of your baby. If you've not had internal examinations, then this is the time from when your body starts to push through to the birth of your baby.

The more relaxed you are, the easier and quicker it will be. As I mentioned, this stage can be anywhere from a couple of minutes through to around the two-hour mark. If your body has been pushing for two hours and baby is not descending, intervention would normally be offered at this point. As with any offer of intervention, you would need to use your B.R.A.I.N. to help you decide what *you* want to do. It might well be the time and place for intervention, and you may be happy to embrace help at this point, or you might prefer to continue as you are. I would suspect that how baby is doing and how you are feeling would be important factors to consider at this point. If you and your baby are tiring then help might be welcomed. If you are both fine, you may be happier to continue as you are for a while longer.

During the second stage or down stage, if all is well you can be confident that you won't be coached to push and will instead be encouraged to listen to your body and go with it by the midwives. If, however, someone did try to coach you unnecessarily or without your permission, your birth partner could step in here and politely ask them to refrain and advocate for you so that your preferences are respected. On that note, I would outline your wishes on your birth preferences document as to how you want to navigate the second stage.

Your down breathing will be a huge help during this stage: a quick inhale through your nose to fill your lungs, then exhaling through your mouth with intent and purpose. Channel your exhale down through your body and feel your muscles respond and move downwards with your breath. Remember to practise this breathing technique on the toilet when going for a poo and get used to the sensation of using your breath as you soften, relax and open to expel something from your body!

It feels like this should be the big finale, but it's not: there's still the third stage to follow.

The third stage of labour (the Golden Hour)

Now on to the 'third stage' of labour, or the forgotten stage. It's easy to assume that once you've birthed your baby, the birth is over. But, actually, the third stage is just as important as the previous stages: it is the birth of the placenta – a very important and essential part of the birth process.

So, timing-wise, the third stage begins when baby is born and ends when the placenta is birthed. This is the length of time that will be recorded in your notes. The placenta is usually birthed within an hour of baby being born, but, equally, it can follow just a few minutes after the baby.

This stage is also known as the 'Golden Hour' because lots of important and magical things happen in the first hour after birth – not all of them visible to the eye – that offer significant benefits for parent and baby.

The key elements of the Golden Hour usually include:

- Immediate skin-to-skin
- Bonding between parent and baby
- Delayed cord clamping
- Delivery of the placenta
- Control of blood loss
- Establishing breastfeeding

Immediate skin-to-skin means placing the baby on to their parent's chest immediately after birth and then leaving them to enjoy some uninterrupted skin-to-skin time. If all is well and nobody requires immediate assistance, they should have uninterrupted skin-to-skin time for the first hour after birth because it offers so many recognised benefits for both parties. If it's not possible for the parent who has given birth to hold the baby for whatever reason, then the baby can enjoy skin-to-skin time with the birth partner. That way, the baby will still get some of the benefits.

Skin-to-skin is recommended best practice after a vaginal birth and you'll find this within the NICE guidelines. This isn't something you should have to request, but just to be sure I always advise stipulating your wishes within your birth preferences document.

Immediate skin-to-skin time, unfortunately, is still not the norm when giving birth in theatre. Times are changing, though, with an increasing number of people requesting natural caesareans, so skin-to-skin in theatre is thankfully becoming more common.

I'm also aware that in some hospitals there are NHS-endorsed posters actively *promoting* skin-to-skin in theatre. But even if it's not the way things are usually done at your hospital or trust, it's always something you can request. And your wishes ought to be respected – especially if you present them in writing, as part of your birth preferences document. Doctors have a legal obligation to respect your wishes because ... it's *your* body, *your* baby, *your* birth and *your* choice! It's very possible to have immediate skin-to-skin time in theatre, so long as parent and baby are both well.

The only time it might not be possible to have immediate and uninterrupted skin-to-skin time with your baby after birth is if you or your baby need immediate medical assistance. But in all other cases, skin-to-skin should be encouraged as soon as possible.

If all is well there is also no need for baby to be weighed, cleaned or assessed within the first hour after birth. Paperwork can wait and your baby won't gain or lose any pounds by deferring the scales for an hour. Likewise, you don't need to be examined, poked, prodded, stitched or washed in the first hour, unless there are urgent medical concerns. Sometimes in a busy labour ward, this Golden Hour can be rushed solely because there's a conveyor belt that needs to keep running, so you need to make sure you stipulate your wishes in writing and your birth partner advocates for you. Ring-fence this time. It can't be got back.

The benefits of skin-to-skin time are numerous, but for baby, who has spent their entire existence thus far listening to the sound of a heartbeat, being placed onto someone's chest at birth can be very reassuring and soothing because although so much of their environment will have changed, they will recognise the familiar sound of the heartbeat and find comfort in that. Skin-to-skin time also initiates the process of bonding for baby.

For the parent who has just given birth the benefits are even more profound. Immediate skin-to-skin time *increases* the production of oxytocin, which, as you know, is your happy, feel-good hormone – the 'love hormone'. Studies have shown that the oxytocin produced at birth helps with bonding, reduces the risk of postnatal depression, reduces the risk of postpartum haemorrhage and increases the success rate of breastfeeding. That's a pretty good list of evidence-based benefits and the main reasons why skin-to-skin time is promoted at birth and recommended in the NICE guidelines.

Oxytocin, as you already know, is a key hormone when it comes to giving birth and plays the important role of fuelling the surges. At the point of birth, you are meant to get a huge rush of oxytocin, which is why so many people describe feeling euphoric and wanting to do it all again. The evolutionary reason for this great rush of oxytocin is so that you immediately bond with your baby, you feel loving and protective towards them, and, as mammals, you don't abandon your vulnerable offspring in the wild, leaving them to fend for themselves!

The other function of oxytocin, apart from making you feel all those things, is that it's the hormone that makes your uterus surge. Even though you have birthed your baby, your uterus muscles still need to work; they need to contract so that the uterus can shrink back down into the pelvis and, by doing so, close off all the open blood vessels where the placenta has detached from the uterus wall, stemming the blood loss. Another evolutionary reason for the oxytocin: we need to stem the blood loss in order to survive and thrive!

So, oxytocin *after* birth is as important as it was during the earlier stages of labour. Being relaxed enables you to produce oxytocin, so everything that was important in the first and second stages of labour is still important now: maintaining a calm environment, feeling informed and confident, relaxed and positive – not feeling fearful or anxious and producing adrenaline. Use your relaxation techniques when (or if) necessary.

Oxytocin also helps with the production of breastmilk. The huge spike in oxytocin is like a message to your milk-making mammaries to say 'Baby has been born! Bring on the milk!' Without the high of oxytocin your breasts may not get the memo. This can cause a delay in your milk coming in and makes getting breastfeeding established more tricky.

All in all, we want *loads* of oxytocin after birth, and skin-to-skin with your new baby is the best way of achieving this. You might consider putting your baby to your breast in this Golden Hour because their latching on and stimulating your breast and nipple will help you produce even more oxytocin. Just as nipple stimulation is sometimes recommended in early labour, putting your baby on your breast achieves the same result post-birth.

The next important element to consider in the Golden Hour is cord clamping. This means clamping and cutting the umbilical cord that joins parent and baby. The choice is either to have the cord clamped and cut straight away, known as immediate cord clamping, or leaving it for a period of time, which is known as delayed cord clamping. Delayed cord clamping means the cord is left intact for *at least* three minutes after the birth. This gives your baby the opportunity to get the majority, if not all, of their blood back.

The reason your baby doesn't have all of their blood inside their body at the point of birth is because, whilst your baby is growing inside your womb, at any given point, approximately a third of their blood is in the placenta. The foetal blood moves continually between the placenta and the baby, transferring vital oxygen and nutrients to the baby as it does so. At the point of birth, a third of your baby's blood is still *in* the placenta! Of course, we know we wouldn't feel too great if we were short-changed a third of our blood, and the same goes for our baby – only they can't tell us how weak and rubbish they feel!

However, by leaving the cord unclamped (delayed cord clamping), the placenta will pump the baby's blood back down the cord, returning it, helpfully, to its rightful owner. If you were to have a look at the umbilical cord after birth, you would *see* this process happening; at birth the cord will be firm, blue (filled with blood) and pulsing. Leaving the cord unclamped for at least three minutes enables the majority of the baby's blood to be returned. Opting for fully delayed cord clamping means leaving the cord intact until *all* the blood has passed through. You will know when this has happened because the cord will be limp, white and visibly empty. This can take up to eight to ten minutes. This might seem like a long time to wait, but, actually, you've just given birth! You're meeting your baby for the first time! You won't notice these initial early minutes passing: they slip by quickly in a blur of overwhelming happiness and delight.

The main reason why delayed cord clamping is recommended – and it's recommended as best practice in the NICE guidelines, which govern NHS practice – is because foetal blood is so rich in goodness. Even though babies who have immediate cord clamping and cutting *can* and *do* compensate by making up the volume of their blood over time, the *quality* of that blood is not the same. Trust that your baby will be just fine if they need to have their cord cut soon after birth – we all probably had our cord cut immediately as that was common practice until recently – but there is evidence to show that it's beneficial (and indeed advantageous) for baby to have all of their blood back where possible. Hence why the NICE guidelines state delayed cord clamping is best practice in vaginal birth.

The next thing to consider in the Golden Hour is a biggie, and that's the delivery of the placenta. You have two options: physiological delivery, which means a natural delivery, or active management, which means drugs are used to manage the process.

Physiological third stage

With a physiological third stage, you birth your baby and wait until all the blood has been pumped back down the cord and returned to the baby (fully delayed cord clamping), you then have the cord clamped and cut, and wait for the placenta to come. Whilst waiting you would be enjoying lovely skin-to-skin time with your newborn baby, taking it all in, revelling in your achievement, so it's unlikely you'd be watching the clock or feeling that it was taking too long.

Waiting for the placenta can take up to an hour after birth, although it can and, often does, come away of its own accord within the first thirty minutes. After an hour, if there's no sign of the placenta coming, the midwives would probably suggest changing to active management – introducing drugs to speed up the process – because the placenta does need to come out. It can't stay in there forever!

If you had given birth in a pool you would be encouraged to step out to birth the placenta on dry land. This is for a number of reasons. Firstly, it's hard for the midwives to gauge blood loss after birth if you're in water: the water can turn red quite quickly, even if you've only lost a small amount of blood. Secondly, it's important your new baby doesn't get cold and if the baby hasn't got its body in the water then they might start to get chilly. Finally, the midwives need to be able to inspect the placenta after birth to check it's all intact. That means making sure it has come away from the uterus wall as a whole and no parts are left inside you. This is difficult to do if the placenta has been birthed into the pool. So, for all these reasons it might be a good idea to step out of the pool once the cord has been cut and perhaps sit on a birth stool if there is one available, cuddling your baby against your chest with the pair of you wrapped in a towel or blanket. Or you could try sitting on the toilet – a good

U.F.O. (upright, forward and open) position which can speed the process up naturally. Or you might like to recline on the sofa if at home (covered in towels/absorbent pads of course!) or the bed if in hospital.

When the placenta does come, you will feel the now-familiar pressure and your body beginning to push. It's *not* like birthing another baby. Equally, it doesn't just slip out unnoticed. Placentas vary in size from person to person, baby to baby, but they tend to be approximately an inch or so thick, and if you place the palms of your hands side by side you'll get an idea of their approximate surface area. So, it's a sizeable organ, which means your body will need to push (you could always use your down breathing again or give a small push yourself) and you'll feel it pass through and then – boom! – you've birthed the placenta and it's the end of the third – and final – stage of labour. *Congratulations!*

What I've just described is a physiological third stage where no drugs are introduced and the placenta is birthed spontaneously. If you've had a straightforward birth, with no intervention, fuelled by your own oxytocin, you're a lot more likely to have a physiological third stage without complication. Oxytocin – that wondrous hormone – is responsible for the uterus shrinking back down after birth, the placenta separating from the uterus wall and being expelled, and then the uterus continuing to contract down, closing off all the open blood vessels where the placenta came away from the uterus wall. The more oxytocin you have in your body, the better! The more oxytocin, the quicker and more straightforward this stage will be.

Active management

Opting for active management changes the pathway of the third stage slightly. With active management you are given a drug to speed up the delivery of the placenta. The drug is given via an injection into your thigh. The cord is usually clamped and cut prior to giving the injection, which *can* interfere with the delayed cord clamping time. The ideal, if you are opting for active management, would be to reach some middle ground where you get a bit of both; your baby has five minutes of delayed cord clamping and the benefits of receiving the majority of their blood back before the cord is cut and you then have active management, which has been shown to reduce the risk of postpartum haemorrhage. However, if there is a medical reason why active management is required (for instance, blood loss), this can dictate how long it would be advisable for the cord clamping to be delayed. Obviously, it's *always* your choice, but if you are losing too much blood you're going to want to get that under control and it would take priority. Untreated, excessive blood loss could potentially be life-threatening, as opposed to immediate cord clamping, which is definitely *not* life-threatening. Delayed cord clamping offers benefits, yes, but if you need immediate cord clamping it's not dangerous for your baby. It can be dangerous, however, if you're losing too much blood after birth. I say this not to scare you, but to recognise the need to be open-minded when outlining your preferences: sometimes things have to change slightly (or even a lot) and that's ok. Understanding why they need to change, opting for what's best for you and your baby and giving informed consent is hugely empowering.

So, how does active management work and why might you opt for it?

The drug you are given for active management is syntocinon – synthetic oxytocin. Oxytocin, as you know, fuels the surges you experience in labour. After birth, although you don't want to experience labour surges again, you *do* want the uterus to contract and shrink back down into your pelvis. Your midwife will check this is happening periodically after birth by placing a hand gently on your abdomen and feeling where the top of your uterus is. As the placenta separates from the uterus wall it leaves a large surface area of open blood vessels, which is where a lot of the blood loss comes from after birth. As the uterus contracts, it closes off these open blood vessels and stems the blood loss. Remember, blood loss after birth is *normal* and to be expected. Normal blood loss is considered to be between 500ml and one litre. A litre is a significant amount of blood, and yet still considered within the parameters of normal loss.

The quicker the uterus contracts and shrinks, the faster those open blood vessels are sealed closed and the blood flow stemmed. Just like with birth, the uterus muscles are fuelled by oxytocin, so the more of it you have, the more effectively (and faster) the uterus muscles will work. Therefore, giving someone an injection of syntocinon (synthetic oxytocin) after birth boosts this natural process, speeds up the delivery of the placenta and gets the blood loss under control faster. For this reason, active management is recommended if you are at an increased risk of experiencing a postpartum haemorrhage.

The three most common reasons (in no particular order) people are offered or opt for active management are:

1. **To speed up the process:** Having the injection is likely to speed up the delivery of the placenta, which you might welcome if you have been in labour for a long time, are exhausted and just want to get into bed with your newborn and a hot cuppa.
2. **To get blood loss under control:** Giving the injection will help the uterus to contract and shrink quicker, closing off the open blood vessels and stemming blood loss. If your midwife thinks you are losing more blood than expected after birth they will recommend active management.

3. Retained placenta: If you have waited an hour and the placenta is showing no signs of coming of its own accord you will be offered the injection. The injection should kick-start the uterus muscles into action and, by contracting, help the placenta separate from the uterus wall.

So, there we have it! All the stages of labour and, most importantly, what actually happens at each stage. Hopefully, having read this chapter, you now feel a lot more informed about how labour (despite its unpredictable nature) *tends* to pan out and the key elements you need to consider when creating your own set of birth preferences.

BIRTH STORY

Positive water birth at an attached birth
centre – Sarah, third-time parent

Baby Wilf was born at thirty-nine weeks and is my third baby. My previous two deliveries were less than ideal, which had left me feeling a bit negative about labour if I'm honest. I had pre-eclampsia with one and a failure to progress with the other, leading to two very 'medical'-feeling births (me on my back, bright lights, lots of bodies, drugs and a total loss of control on my part).

Wilf's birth could not have been more different and I am still on Cloud Nine about how well it went. I feel the whole delivery was a testament to hypnobirthing. On the morning of the birth I just knew he was on his way and I was excited about what would happen next, rather than anxious. I had my eldest son's nativity play at the local church at 10am, and by the time I was sitting down listening to him singing I was having light surges every fifteen minutes or so. Back at home, they continued in the same manner for the best part of the day and I chilled out, watching The Holiday, drinking tea and eating biscuits.

At 4pm, I attempted a nap to bank some sleep and help me to relax but found I could no longer sleep through the surges, which were around every ten minutes. Then, at 5pm, my waters broke all over the living room floor (proper comedy waters gush like in the movies – it was everywhere). It was at this point that I had a bit of a worry as I realised, with all the excitement over things happening, that I hadn't felt the baby move for a couple of hours. After phoning triage at the hospital, I was told to come in just to check the baby's heart rate and, although I had hoped to relax at home for a lot longer to minimise hospital time (my chosen birthplace was the birth centre at the hospital rather than the labour ward), I needed peace of mind, so we loaded the car with the hospital bags and headed off.

His heart rate was fine, but it was at this point that I really feared my birth plan was about to fly out the window as my blood pressure reading was sky high and, given my history of pre-eclampsia, this was a big concern. After consultation with doctors, the midwives told me that the advice was to send me to the labour ward and not the birth centre, and that a water birth was not recommended due to an increased risk of fitting associated with my blood pressure. I asked questions about risks and benefits (needing to change my mindset about 'not being allowed' to do things) and, given that I was now having surges every two minutes, asked if it would be possible to get into a pool at the birth centre and reassess my blood pressure there, as I had a feeling that the baby would be making an appearance very soon and feared the labour ward would set me back. The midwives were brilliant and, given that my blood pressure was not yet an emergency situation, they agreed to try it my way for a bit in the hope that the pool would relax me. I was relieved beyond belief and within half an hour I was in the pool.

The next two hours were everything I'd hoped birth would be this time around. My husband, James, put some gentle spa music on, we sprayed the Liquid Yoga room spray and I went into my own zone, focusing on breathing and, lo and behold, my blood pressure went down, hurrah! For an hour and a half, I barely made any noise except to breathe (I can't tell you how different this was to my second birth, where I swore, shouted and cried!) and I really made use of the visualisation techniques, particularly the hot-air balloon one.

James kept offering me water and sweets between surges to keep my strength up and sat by my side the whole time, which definitely made it feel like my safe space. At around 11.25pm I felt like things had changed and that the up breathing was no longer working with me, like something was pushing down into my bottom. I knew it was time to change to the down breaths. Despite having had no internal examinations, my body knew that it was time for him to arrive.

After twenty minutes using the blowing-out-candle breaths, his head was out (again, I felt so calm, stopping to have a chat about the colour of his hair!) and then shortly after, with one final big surge the rest of him followed just before midnight. The cord was wrapped twice around his neck which made me panic momentarily but he was absolutely fine and the midwife helped me to get him onto my chest. The feeling at that point was total euphoria and I felt like a superhero – I have never been prouder of myself, and after two pretty negative births I almost felt like this birth had put the others right somehow. He was 8lb 13oz – my biggest baby yet – but I had paracetamol and codeine only, not even gas and air this time as I just didn't feel like I wanted them (I've sampled all the drugs in previous births and never enjoyed the sensation of being 'out of it'). Post-birth, things almost got medical again when the placenta got stuck and had to be manually manipulated out by the midwife, but, again, I breathed through it and the atmosphere was not one of panic. After tea and toast, some skin-to-skin and the first feed we left the hospital just a few hours later and were back at home by 5am, meaning our older two had gone to bed like normal and woken up to find a baby sibling!

I think the reason this birth was so different was due to the preparation I put in and the resulting conviction I had in my own decisions.

9

Bring it on, baby! Induction

Induction is a fairly common procedure in the UK with around 20 per cent of births being induced each year. In this chapter I will go through why you might opt for an induction, what an induction typically entails and, finally, how you can ensure a positive experience using your hypnobirthing toolkit. Lots of people ask me if hypnobirthing can still help and be used if they are being induced and I always say that the tools you will learn are even *more* powerful when things become more challenging or complex. There is no scenario in which your toolkit will not help.

I believe it's important to discuss induction in detail, partly because so many pregnancies are induced, but mainly because I believe that if people understand what the full induction pathway looks like they will be better prepared if they opt for this route, and less likely to be taken by surprise. When speaking to people who have experienced birth trauma, common themes include not understanding what was happening and feeling out of control. Much of this can be avoided by ensuring you fully understand the choices you are making.

Given that induction is discussed routinely at your forty-week midwife appointment – and the vast majority of people will still be pregnant at forty weeks – chances are you will, at the very least, be having a conversation about induction. Unfortunately, the time you get with your midwife at routine appointments is generally quite limited, and so, too, is the scope to discuss all elements of birth in detail. The result is that many people go into birth and induction without knowing what to expect. This chapter aims to remedy that. By leaving you more informed, you will feel a lot more relaxed when induction is brought up in discussion, as well as confident that, should you opt for one, you can make it a positive, empowering and happy experience.

Why might you opt for an induction?

Reasons for offering an induction vary: from waters breaking and labour not beginning, to repeated episodes of reduced movement, or developing a medical condition such as gestational diabetes, pre-eclampsia, obstetric cholestasis, and so on. The most common reason, however, is down to dates: being considered 'overdue'. Given that the estimated due date is just that – an estimate – it might come as a surprise that so many people are going down the route of induction based on due dates alone. [11]

Opting for induction is not a decision to be taken lightly. I have mentioned already my own experience, but will reiterate again that I didn't know of any risks associated with induction when agreeing to my own induction of labour. I beat myself up for years believing that it was because I was young and naive at the time, but, having spoken to hundreds of other people since, I know that I am not alone in my experience and that it had nothing to do with my age. People are being induced every day without fully realising a) what's involved b) what the risks are, and c) without realising that it is *their choice*.

How many times have you heard someone say: 'They won't let me go past forty-one weeks', for example? They won't *let* you? Are medical professionals really going to come and physically drag you from your home and hook you up to an IV drip against your will? No! Of course, they can't do that. Nobody can force you to have an induction – at any stage in your pregnancy. *It is always your choice.* Naturally, there are guidelines and they exist for a reason (and in many cases it would be wise to follow them), but you are under no obligation to do so. Remember, these are guidelines created for the entire population; they are not bespoke to you or your baby.

Sometimes, unfortunately, you may feel as though you *are* being told what to do and that you *don't* have a choice, but it's at that exact moment that you most need to engage your B.R.A.I.N. What you are being told is only ever advice or a recommendation, never a direct order. If a medical professional says they 'won't let you' go past such and such a date, I'd be tempted to gently remind them that *you* will be making the decision as to when – or even *if* – you will agree to an induction. Remember: *your* body, *your* baby, *your* birth and *your* choice! *Always.*

With regard to the induction of labour, proving it's never a decision to be taken lightly, the NICE guidelines state:

> Induced labour has an impact on the birth experience of women. It may be less efficient and is usually more painful than spontaneous labour, and epidural analgesia and assisted delivery are more likely to be required [...] Induction of labour has a large impact on the health of women and their babies and so needs to be clearly clinically justified.[12]

The guidelines clearly acknowledge that induction has a (not particularly positive-sounding) impact on the *experience* of birth itself and a large impact on the *health* of those giving birth and their babies. I am certainly not at any point advocating that you decline all offers of induction and resist all intervention (or even perceive intervention to be always a negative thing!), but rather I encourage you to reflect on the evidence-based guidelines produced by NICE and the information available, taking all this into consideration when making your decision.

The NICE guidelines recognise that induction leads to an increase in the risk of intervention, assisted delivery and the need for an epidural. This makes it clear that it is not a decision to be taken lightly. In fact, the entire guidelines on induction make for an interesting read, especially if you're considering opting for one. I'd urge you to read the guidelines in full as a necessity if an induction has been offered.

Parking the increase in risks for a moment, what really stands out in the statement is that it 'needs to be clearly clinically justified'. This to me is the most important part of the whole statement. Is the offer of induction *clearly clinically justified*? To *you*?

If it's not, then the brakes need to be swiftly applied! You're going to need more information: use your B.R.A.I.N., ask the relevant questions and establish whether induction is the right course of action for you and your baby. Take into consideration the known risks, have a look at the supposed benefits and then ask yourself: do the benefits outweigh the risks? Consider the alternatives, which include expectant management and additional monitoring, and listen to your instinct, asking yourself: what feels right for me? Also ask what would happen if you were to take some time to consider everything, or even postpone an induction. Would there be any potential negative consequences in doing so? And, finally, ask to *see* the clinical justification! Can the doctor or midwife show you, or at least point you in the direction of the study in which the outcome clearly shows that for you and your situation, induction is the best course of action compared to any alternatives or expectant management. If there is no evidence, if none exists, then it's *not clearly clinically justified*. It's just someone's opinion. And you can always ask for a second opinion. But at the end of the day, the *only* opinion that really matters is yours because it's your choice.

So, what counts as 'clinical justification'? Clinical justification might include, but is certainly not limited to:

- Waters breaking and labour not beginning spontaneously – the waters protect the baby from bumps, keep the baby warm and also protect the baby from any bacteria travelling up into the uterus. Once the waters around the baby have released, they no longer have that protection and therefore the risk of infection starts to rise. The advice varies from hospital to hospital, but most are keen to induce between twenty-four and forty-eight hours after waters releasing if there's no sign of labour beginning. This is a clinically justified reason because it's known that the risk of infection increases for both the expectant parent and their unborn baby.
- Gestational diabetes, pre-eclampsia and obstetric cholestasis are medical conditions that can develop in pregnancy. These conditions *can* pose a serious threat to the well-being of those who are pregnant and their babies and therefore can be considered as clinically justified reasons for an induction being offered. The severity of these conditions can vary and, of course, might influence your final decision.
- Dates: prolonged pregnancy is a term used to describe a pregnancy lasting longer than forty-two weeks and is the most common reason for induction. According to the World Health Organisation, if someone is between

thirty-seven and forty-two weeks pregnant, they are perfectly within their due period and not a single day overdue or late. After forty-two weeks, however, you are considered to have gone beyond your due period and can therefore be considered post-term or 'overdue'. But, crucially, not *before* forty-two weeks!

We have a (bad) habit here in the UK of talking about being 'overdue' and 'late' as soon as we go a single day past our given estimated due date, although it's known that fewer than 5 per cent of babies are born *on* their due date, meaning a whopping 95 per cent of babies aren't! What's more, the majority of those babies are being born after their due date, rather than before (almost 75 per cent of babies are born after their due date at forty weeks).[13]

The estimated due date is extremely unreliable as an indicator of when your baby is actually likely to be born, yet so many people form their plans around, and pin all their expectations on, this one single date. This can cause a lot of disappointment and frustration.

In terms of prolonged pregnancy and induction, the reason the latter is offered is because there is evidence to show that the risk of stillbirth rises slowly after thirty-eight weeks. Interestingly, the risk of stillbirth throughout the pregnancy decreases as time goes on until it reaches the lowest point between thirty-seven and thirty-eight weeks, at which point it starts to rise again. So, the risk of stillbirth post-thirty-eight weeks is not dissimilar to the risk that existed prior to thirty-eight weeks. You're not at an *increased* risk in comparison to earlier points in your pregnancy. If you plotted the results on a graph you would see a U shape. After forty weeks the risk continues to rise, but we are still talking about a very low risk overall. The risk of stillbirth goes from 0.4 in 1000 at forty weeks to 0.6

in 1000 at forty-one weeks.[14] It might be a 50 per cent increase in terms of *relative* risk, but we are still talking about very small numbers – four people in 10,000 to six people in 10,000. This is the main reason why the NHS prefers all babies to be born by forty-two weeks, but the absolute risk remains low.

Introducing routine induction at forty-one weeks might prevent two babies out of 10,000 being stillborn, but – and it's a big but – if *everyone* was induced at forty-one weeks, then 9,994 babies (and their parents) would be subjected to the increased risks associated with induction unnecessarily. And, as the NICE guidelines clearly state, induction has an impact on the birth experience, may be less effective, is usually more painful and increases the risk of intervention, including assisted delivery and the need for an epidural.

After forty-two weeks, when you are considered post-term, the risk increases to 10 in 10,000 (or 1 in 1000).[15] This may well count as clinical justification, but, remember, it is *still* your choice. There are also increased risks to you and your baby's health by accepting an induction. Unfortunately, as much as we wish there was, there is no guaranteed, absolute risk-free option when it comes to giving birth. You need to weigh up the options you have, take into account your situation and make your own informed decision. Nobody else can make it for you! So, use your B.R.A.I.N. and ask yourself: which seems the best course of action for me? You may well reach a different decision to somebody else (which is more than fine: there is no right or wrong when it comes to giving birth!). We are diverse, autonomous individuals and we will birth and raise our children in different ways, and that is something to be celebrated.

It's worth knowing that post forty-two weeks you have the right to opt for increased antenatal monitoring. If you're using your B.R.A.I.N., this would be the 'A' for Alternative answered. So, you have the Benefits of induction for dates – reducing the risk of stillbirth associated with prolonged pregnancy; the Risks – increased risk of intervention, assisted delivery, epidural; and the Alternative – increased antenatal monitoring and expectant management. Now you need to check in with your instinct – what does that tell you? And ask what happens if you do Nothing for twenty-four hours and come back the next morning?

Perhaps you want to do some research of your own to understand the other risk factors for stillbirth, and maybe that will help inform your decision. For example, having a BMI over thirty increases the risk, so if that applies to you, you might veer towards accepting an induction. However, if you are 'low-risk' and enjoying a straightforward pregnancy, you *might* feel more confident opting for increased antenatal monitoring.

I'm not advocating one option over another. I'm definitely not advocating that you decline induction no matter what. What's important to me is that you know you have options and you are able to make an informed decision as to which one is best for you. There is no right or wrong answer, and it wouldn't be for me to decide in any case. I'm drawing upon a few examples that could apply to you and which you might wish to consider, but by no means am I comprehensively covering *all* potential scenarios. However, you get the gist: whatever your scenario, use your B.R.A.I.N. and make sure you understand the clear clinical justification for the induction before you consider accepting.

Remember, at the beginning of this book I said there's a time and a place for everything, including intervention. It might well be the case that this *is* the time and the place for you, in which case you want to be able to embrace this new pathway. But if it's not the time or the place for you, then you want to feel confident knowing that you can decline.

I am absolutely not advocating that you decline all intervention. I want to make that really clear. In fact, quite the opposite! I want you to *embrace* necessary intervention and have a positive birth experience where you feel calm and assured! But most of all I want to encourage you to use your B.R.A.I.N. so that, as you navigate your pregnancy and birth, you'll know when to accept and embrace, and equally when to feel confident declining. I believe using the B.R.A.I.N. framework to get the information you need to make informed choices will help massively, whether in terms of induction or anything else.

Most importantly, by making your own decision (even, or *especially,* when that decision is in agreement with what has been suggested), you can feel strong, capable and in control – which is exactly how you want to feel when you welcome your baby into the world. Remember, the mechanics of *how* your baby enters the world matter little long-term in comparison to *how you felt* when your baby came into the world. This is an enormous life-changing moment, whether it's your first or your fourth, and so I really encourage you to take charge, ask questions, challenge people if necessary and make your own decision. It's not about declining intervention or being anti-intervention; it's about understanding why the intervention is being offered and knowing whether it's the right thing for you, or not. If it's the right thing, then great! We can be thankful that the option is there. That is a big positive.

Here are some examples of things that don't count as clinical justification (but which have been known to have been given as reasons for induction):

- Christmas is soon
- It's quiet on the ward today
- Baby's size

The first one might surprise you – you're thinking *Surely not!* – but it actually happens quite a bit. If you know anyone who had a baby around Christmas, ask them if they encountered this.

The last one might surprise you, because it seems like a relatively plausible reason for an induction, doesn't it? Because, what if the baby *is* too big? Is it not better to get them out sooner rather than later? Before they grow even bigger! Well, as surprising as it might be, there is actually no firm evidence to say that inducing someone because their baby measures big significantly improves the overall outcomes for them or their baby. In the absence of gestational diabetes, the (low) risk of shoulder dystocia (where the baby's head is born but the shoulder becomes stuck) is the same for big and small babies. Yet we know that opting for induction *increases* a number of risks. The NICE guidelines back this up and confirm that in the absence of any other indications, induction should not be carried out simply because it's suspected that the baby is large for their gestational age.[16]

Also worth remembering if you are told your baby is measuring big (or small) is that the scans which are used to determine the size of a baby are not 100 per cent accurate and that the later on in the pregnancy you are, and the bigger the baby, the more difficult it is to get an accurate estimate of the size or weight of the baby. That's why the NICE guidelines state that size alone should not be a factor for induction. Size of baby, coupled with something like gestational diabetes, could justify offering an induction.

Finally, on the topic of size, nobody can tell you that your baby is *too* big for your body. Our bodies are truly incredible things and when you are in labour, you will have high levels of relaxin in your body, softening all the tissue, muscles and ligaments. Everything will be soft and stretchy. Your pelvis will widen to accommodate baby and your coccyx will move out of the way! Your baby's head will then decrease in size (the four plates of a baby's skull being able to overlap one another) to perfectly fit within the space available. I have known many people who are very petite go on to birth 9lb or 10lb babies without any assistance and without suffering even a small tear. Your body is capable of birthing your baby. And, in some cases, bigger can be better! I have heard midwives say that big babies can speed up a labour, descending faster because the extra weight on the cervix helps it to open; a nice big baby also stretches the vaginal walls effectively during their descent. It's actually very small, pre-term babies who are more likely to require assistance being born.

What does an induction typically entail?

What happens if you use your B.R.A.I.N. and decide that there *is* enough clinical justification and good reason to agree to an induction? Now you want to be able to embrace it. So, what does the process actually entail?

Induction can begin in different ways for different people and varies depending on the reason for the induction in the first place. Most people, however, will initially be offered a prostaglandin pessary or gel. Prostaglandin is a hormone that ripens the cervix and helps it to thin (efface) and open (dilate).

A pessary is similar to a mini tampon and it is inserted up into the vagina and positioned at the opening of the cervix. The gel is applied internally around the cervix. Both work in a similar way. You will usually be left for six hours and then re-examined. If there is little to no change then you can have a second pessary and again wait another six hours. It's possible, after monitoring the baby and if all is well, for you to go home during these six hours and, when possible, it's probably a good idea. Just like with natural labour, you want to be as relaxed as possible so you can release the necessary oxytocin and work *with* the pessary. This will give you the best chance of going into labour. So, consider what will help you relax. Will it be remaining on the main, noisy, busy labour ward, sitting on a hospital bed in a small bay with the curtains pulled around you, strip lights on and listening to the conversations of those in other bays? Probably not. Go home if you can, dim the lights, snuggle up on the sofa, watch something funny on the TV, have a bath, have a rest, practise your relaxation. If you can't go home, maybe try and go for a walk around the hospital grounds. Whatever it is you do, aim to relax. If you do need to stay on the main ward, wear an eye mask and your comfiest clothes, spritz your scented room spray and use some headphones to get in the zone. The more relaxed you are, the more likely things are to get going.

In the best-case scenario, the pessary alone will work. That would be excellent! If there are no medical concerns (perhaps you opted for induction based on dates) then, in theory, you could now go home and have the home birth you wanted, or a water birth or whatever it is you were originally planning. If the pessary or gel works and you're in established labour and all is well with you and baby, then little has to change. Your original birth preferences can be followed and you don't have to deviate.

However, if the pessaries or gel don't work, then the next step is to break your waters (called artificial rupture of membranes – ARM) and to use syntocinon (synthetic oxytocin), which is administered via a drip to get the surges going. At this point things will step up a notch and a few elements of your original birth preferences may need to change.

For example, you will need to be on the labour ward for the syntocinon drip – this can't be given at home or in a midwife-led unit or birth centre. Your waters need to be broken before the syntocinon is administered, and it's advised that you have continuous monitoring as opposed to intermittent monitoring – the latter being more usual when things are unfolding in a straightforward way. Continuous monitoring means having two wide elastic bands fitted around your abdomen keeping two monitors in place. These monitors pick up the surges and your baby's heartbeat and are usually attached by wires (although some hospitals have a wireless option) to a machine that prints out the information, making it easier for doctors and midwives to keep a close eye on how your baby is doing throughout. Continuous monitoring can be restrictive, certainly more so than intermittent monitoring, which is when a midwife listens in every so often to check on baby's well-being using a handheld doppler device. However, continuous monitoring is recommended when being induced with syntocinon as it's recognised that this type of induction increases the risk of baby experiencing distress.

In most cases, you will be advised that it's no longer possible to use a birth pool due to the need for continuous monitoring. However, remember who is in charge: it's *you*! And if being in the water is important to you, and we know it offers benefits including comfort and relaxation, then you can state that you wish to use a pool (as long as one is available) and ask the doctors or midwives providing your care how they can facilitate that. Very rarely is a 'no' a hard no. Sometimes it's a no because that's not what's usually done. But you can step off that conveyor belt at any point and push for the birth *you* want. There is always room for negotiation and your preferences must be respected; you call the shots!

If you do opt for the pool, you would still have your waters broken and the syntocinon would still be administered by a drip, but you would need to keep your arm out of the water. You can always have a waterproof dressing applied to cover the cannula fitting, protecting it from getting wet. And then you would likely have frequent monitoring by a midwife using a handheld doppler, which can go under the water and be used in the pool. Of course, you might not be that bothered about using a pool, but if you are then it is still possible.

There is a noticeable difference in the level of intervention between an induction with a pessary or gel and an induction on the syntocinon drip. It's unfortunately impossible at the outset of an induction to know whether the pessary will work for you, or whether you will need to progress to have the drip. If only one could know! This is why it's important to know what the full pathway looks like, so you know what you are consenting to. I have heard from many people who told me they agreed to a pessary because it sounded straightforward and meant they could still give birth in the birth centre but had no idea what would happen if the pessary didn't work. They were therefore shocked when just a few hours later they found themselves on a busy labour ward having their waters broken and being strapped up to monitors on a bed, feeling a million miles away from the birth they had anticipated. So much of this shock or even trauma could be avoided if people were properly informed, understood what they were consenting to and had an accurate expectation or understanding of what lay ahead.

When teaching classes I often get asked at this point: if you're calling the shots, can you opt for a pessary but, if that doesn't work, choose not to have the syntocinon drip? And it's a very good question.

In theory, *yes*! You could opt for the pessary and change your mind at any point. You could decline the syntocinon drip if the pessary didn't work. But … in reality, there's probably a good reason for you having consented to induction in the first place. Hopefully you established what the clear clinical justification was before having the pessary inserted. So, if that pessary doesn't work, you're still left with whatever the original issue was. The issue has not been resolved and therefore presumably there is still a clear, clinically justified reason for induction. It would therefore probably be in your best interests to either continue with the induction or opt for a caesarean if you believe that would be better for you and your baby.

BIRTH STORY

Induction (with drip) – Elinor, first-time parent

I was diagnosed with gestational diabetes at thirty weeks and had been planning a home birth. However, even though it was diet controlled, the baby started measuring big on scans. Really big. I started having quite intense meetings with consultants about delivery and interventions and started to feel like I was losing control of the situation. We began asking lots of questions and practising the breathing techniques at home.

At thirty-seven weeks baby was measuring 9lb 6oz and they were advising us to induce straight away. Using B.R.A.I.N. we decided (after reviewing our own personal medical situation) that we wanted to wait. Baby was fine, apart from size, but we really had to push our case. We had extra monitoring and went up to the due date. At forty weeks and one day the consultant said he was pretty much guaranteed to be 12lb 6oz (a worrying thought for a first-time parent!) so we decided to induce the following day. When we arrived I was already 2cm, so they broke my waters and gave me a few hours before starting the drip.

The drip was intense. I knew it would be and this is when the hypnobirthing course kicked in fully! My husband Erik was incredible. He set up the room with lights, music, smells and set about counting and telling me calm, loving stuff to relax me between each surge.

There was a brief moment when I felt I lost control: in the second stage I was down breathing and remembering all the scary meetings and doctors telling me I should have a C-section, and I basically lost faith in myself. Again, Erik was amazing and used all of his course practice to help me remember what I was doing and why. The midwife was incredible and focused on using the words we'd requested until the very last surge where baby got slightly stuck and she said: 'Just put a push behind your next breath' (as the baby was struggling).

Our baby arrived after four hours on the syntocinon drip and afterwards I couldn't believe I'd done it! The breathing is massive, especially for induction I think; it keeps you going. Also I used the mantras 'bring on the next surge' and 'each surge brings me closer to my baby' in the gaps. Having Erik know the course so thoroughly kept him focused and calm even when it got a bit rushed at the end. The birth preferences template was followed by our midwife to the letter and Erik got to tell me it was a baby boy which was so special.

And after all that ... he was a 'huge' 8lb 8oz.

How to use your hypnobirthing toolkit to ensure a positive experience

Now that you know what's involved in an induction, I want you to revisit the initial statement from the NICE guidelines: 'Induced labour has an impact on the birth experience of women. It may be less efficient and is usually more painful than spontaneous labour, and epidural analgesia and assisted delivery are more likely to be required.'[17]

Let's consider for a moment what induction *could* look like if we did not have our toolkit. Someone would be on labour ward (which as you know feels very clinical if you don't make any changes), they may well be reclined on a bed, wearing a hospital gown, sitting on an incontinence pad having had their waters broken, and hooked up to a drip for the syntocinon and monitors to track their baby's heartbeat. All the main lights could be on and people might be coming and going.

It's obvious that very little in this scenario would help the person relax, and the chances are that they would fall quickly into the negative fear → tension → pain cycle we previously discussed – the consequences of which are that their labour becomes less efficient and more painful. If labour is less efficient and someone is reclined on a bed, the risk of intervention becoming necessary increases, and if labour becomes more painful the chances of the person requesting pain relief also increase. Does this sound familiar?

I really believe it's not the syntocinon that directly increases the need for an epidural or assisted delivery. It's not the induction itself that makes labour less efficient and more painful; rather, in most cases, I would suggest that it's the whole package that comes with it – everything I described above – that impacts the labour.

But all that can be changed. You can transform the environment, adopt a good U.F.O. position and use your toolkit to remain calm and relaxed so that you produce oxytocin and everything works efficiently and comfortably.

If you've had a negative experience of induction from a previous birth (as I did back in 2007) I want you to know that your next birth *can* and *will* be different, even if it's induced again.

Firstly, no two births are ever the same – even if you try to repli-
cate exactly everything you did the first time. But secondly, you
are going to do enough things so differently that it would be
impossible for your birth experience to be the same. So, rather
than be concerned about history repeating itself, I want you to
read on and find out what you can do differently if you opt for
induction again. I also hope that reading the above helps you
to make sense of what happened to you previously and why. I
hope it helps you to understand your previous experience – why
things happened the way they did – and leaves you feeling even
more confident about your upcoming birth.

People often ask me: 'But can I still do hypnobirthing if
I'm being induced?' and the answer is *yes*! Nobody really
does hypnobirthing anyway – it's merely a programme of
antenatal education that you can follow as you prepare for
birth. But in terms of *using* the hypnobirthing relaxation
techniques, absolutely *yes*! There's no situation where being
relaxed won't help in birth. And when it comes to induction,
and birth becoming potentially more complex or challenging, it's even more important to have a set of tools that you
can use to help you stay calm in order to navigate your birth
confidently and make informed decisions. If birth is easy and
straightforward, that's wonderful! But when birth is more
challenging – that's when these tools come into a world of
their own. So yes, use all of what you've learnt throughout
the induction process.

By doing so, you will ensure you are working *with* the syntocinon drip and not against it, giving your body and the induction
the best chance of doing their amazing thing. I do believe this is
key when having an induction. You want to be able to produce
your own oxytocin alongside the synthetic version you're being
given so you feel good and the surges you experience are effective and remain comfortable. Natural oxytocin has so many

benefits (including aiding bonding, establishing breastfeeding, reducing blood loss, reducing the risk of postnatal depression and so on) and you can reap the rewards of this by being in a relaxed and happy state of mind. Plus, the more oxytocin you produce, the more likely labour is to unfold quickly, easily and comfortably.

How's that going to happen if you opt for induction and you need the syntocinon drip? Here's how: first of all, you're going to walk into that room and you're going to set the scene for the birth you want! Using your five senses as a checklist you're going to transform what could be a clinical-looking space into a calm and tranquil, spa-like space! Think lighting, sound, smell. Perhaps you're going to put out some battery-operated tea lights or fairy lights, but definitely switch off the main lights! Maybe you're going to play spa music or similar, soothing background music. Perhaps you've made a playlist or are going to listen to your guided relaxations or positive affirmations. Perhaps you have a room spray, some essential oils or a diffuser. Whatever it is you've packed, get the bits out now and set the scene. Remember, never underestimate the impact of the environment: make sure it works for you and that everything in it is going to aid your relaxation.

Next, you're going to have your waters broken. For this you may well lie down on the bed for ease and comfort, but you do not have to wear a hospital gown. You may be in a hospital but you're not a patient and you're not poorly: you're going to have a baby! So, wear something comfortable and cosy – or something cool if you're too warm.

Once your waters have been broken you will want to get up onto your feet and remain mobile. How are you going to do this if your waters are leaking? Easy! How will you manage after birth? You'll wear a pad. You should have some big, absorbent maternity pads in your birth bag, along with some big comfy pants. Pop them on! Now you can remain mobile and upright, wearing your own comfy clothes.

Now baby will need to be monitored, and it's likely that you'll be offered continuous monitoring. It's always worth asking if the hospital has a wireless monitor, because if it does that will give you even more freedom. But if it doesn't, fear not! You can still remain upright and mobile, even if attached by wires to the machine. Yes, you might not have the full freedom of movement you would if you weren't being continuously monitored, but you can still stand up and sway from side to side holding on to the foot of the bed or the sink in the room, you can still pace should you want to move, and you can certainly sit on a birth ball whilst being monitored. All of these positions ensure you're upright, forward and open and make for an easier and quicker birth.

Now perhaps it's time to administer the syntocinon, so you're going to have a cannula fitted. Hopefully the surges will soon start coming and building in strength – this is what you want to happen! So, what are you going to do now? You – with your birth partner's support, ideally – are going to open up that metaphorical toolbox and start using all of the hypnobirthing tools that you have learnt and been practising; you're going to breathe through the surges, in for four, out for eight, with your birth partner counting for you and coaching you through each one, and then you're going to rest and relax in between. Don't forget to drink and eat if you can. It's important to stay hydrated and well fuelled as this helps your muscles work to their full potential. Don't forget that you can use any of the relaxation techniques *between* the surges to help you to let go of any tension and relax further. For example, arm stroking or light-touch massage. In fact, there is no hypnobirthing tool that won't work with induction.

So just to recap, if you're going for an induction you're going to:

- Make the environment work for you, using your five senses as a checklist. You're going to transform the space into a romantic, candlelit room, which smells and sounds like a spa.
- You're going to wear comfortable clothes and remain mobile, adopting U.F.O. positions.
- You're going to eat your yummy treats and stay hydrated.
- You're going to use all of your hypnobirthing toolkit to remain calm and relaxed throughout each surge and in between.
- And you're going to produce loads of oxytocin and most importantly, *feel like an absolute superhero!*

Soon enough, you will be fully dilated and then you're ready to move into the down stage. You can find a great U.F.O. position in which you feel most comfortable and you're going to use your down breathing, with gravity on your side, to breathe your baby down and out. Your body is going to work as it is designed to and your uterus muscles are going to push powerfully downwards with each surge. You will feel your baby descending – the most incredible feeling – and you're going to know that very, very soon you will be holding your baby in your arms.

With the help of your birth partner, you're going to be calm and focused and your body is going to do its amazing thing and you are going to keep on breathing through each surge so your baby is born gently and calmly, just as you wanted.

If you have gravity on your side and you're relaxed, allowing everything to soften and open as your baby descends, then you're giving your body the best chance of doing its job without assistance. *You are doing it!*

And then your baby will be here and you will feel *amazing!* Euphoric! Like a superhero! Because you know that you're the incredible person who just had an induction and made it the positive and empowering birth experience that you wanted.

Pain relief

Hypnobirthing is not about giving birth without pain relief, although everything you'll learn in this book will make your birth more comfortable. Being relaxed is absolutely key – the more relaxed you are, the more comfortable it will be – and your toolkit (and practice!) will help you access a place of deep relaxation.

That said, pain relief exists for a reason. If you are experiencing pain, for whatever reason, and you are suffering, then the experience is no longer positive. The hypnobirthing programme I teach aims to help expectant parents have *positive* birth experiences. It's not about encouraging people to suffer through their birth experience without pain relief in the hope of receiving some sort of medal. There's a big difference.

But equally I don't actively advocate that people use pain relief, because each form of pain relief carries with it its own set of risks – as well as benefits. Like with everything in birth, I encourage people to be informed about their options, so they can make the right decision for them and their baby.

For example, gas and air (also known as laughing gas) can work well, as it can be used with up breathing by inhaling through the mouthpiece rather than your nose. It doesn't pass to the baby, you can still use a pool and adopt a U.F.O. position, and because you can still feel what's happening you won't need to be coached to push – but the downside is that it makes some people feel nauseous and out of control.

Another option is an epidural, which is brilliant in that it provides complete relief, but the downside is that you will usually be constrained to lying on a bed afterwards (although not always). This can slow down labour and restrict your pelvis from opening to its full potential, which increases your risk of experiencing a tear or requiring intervention.

What's most important when it comes to pain relief is knowing that you do have options and no one should have to suffer in birth. Hopefully this is a reassuring thought!

Finally, it's true that many people – myself included – find that the hypnobirthing techniques are so effective they don't need any pain relief at all. However, there are also many people who do choose to have pain relief. There's no right or wrong here! Every person, every baby and every birth is different. The good news is that you can continue to use all of your hypnobirthing toolkit – and everything you learn in this book – alongside all of the forms of pain relief.

BIRTH STORY

Induction (with pessary) – Paige, second-time parent

At my routine midwife appointment, when I had reached forty-one weeks pregnant, I was offered induction for the Saturday of that week, which I decided to decline. After using my B.R.A.I.N. I decided that I would prefer to wait an extra couple of days and get to a full forty-two weeks before induction to give my body the best chance of going into labour spontaneously. Yet Monday morning (at a full forty-two weeks) arrived with still no sign of baby, so it was time to make the phone call to the hospital to arrange a time for me to go in for induction.

We arrived on the maternity unit at the hospital that morning at 11am, and by lunchtime I had been monitored, examined and given a pessary in the hope of getting things moving. The midwife told us that I would need to be monitored again at 6pm that evening and encouraged Ben and I to go out for a walk and enjoy the sunshine in the meantime, so we did exactly that. By the time 6pm arrived I was having irregular surges again, which continued to grow in intensity until we got to around midnight, at which point they were around four minutes apart and very intense. I had been managing just by using my up breathing, my TENS machine and watching a funny film on Netflix to keep myself occupied. Meanwhile, Ben was keeping track of every surge with the help of our pregnancy app. A midwife examined me again and to my delight I was almost 4cm dilated. She offered to take us up to the delivery suite to have my waters broken in the hope of speeding things along, to which I agreed.

I was absolutely elated to arrive at the delivery suite to find that the midwife who took care of me throughout my first pregnancy was on duty. She recognised Ben and I straight away. She took us into a room and we had a chat and I told her of my dream to have a water birth. She told me that the birth pool room was available and that it would be good for me, setting a positive tone, if she were to take us straight in and get us settled there instead. I have never been so grateful to anyone for anything, and I can safely say that just being in the same room as the pool, and having such a wonderful midwife with us, made me completely relaxed and at ease, as if my dream water birth really was still within reach.

Ben set the scene for us by dimming the lighting, spraying our Liquid Yoga room spray and playing my favourite spa music. My midwife broke my waters at 1.40am and as soon as I stood up afterwards I knew things had changed. My surges were coming thicker and faster than ever – every one to two minutes – and the intensity was at a definite peak. I asked for some gas and air but quickly decided this wasn't helping and only made me feel less in control. I told my midwife that she needed to start running the pool as I felt things were happening quickly. By the time I was able to get in I already felt that something had changed – I had reached the down stage. I told her that I felt like I needed to push but thought I might hurt myself; it had only been a very short time ago that she had told me I was 3–4cm dilated. However, she reassured me that some people dilate very quickly and to trust my body and go with it. I found the transition quite overwhelming, but I'm proud to say it was the only time throughout my entire labour that I had a little wobble for a few minutes. Ben soon got me back down in the green zone with some words of encouragement and positive affirmations.

By this point our lovely birth photographer had arrived and asked how I was doing. I shouted: 'The baby is coming! The baby is coming!', along with some animal-like sounds that I had no idea I was capable of making. Ben joined me in the pool in his boxers as instructed and after only a couple of pushes I could feel our baby's head being born – one of the most incredible sensations I have ever felt. I can honestly say I felt no discomfort and certainly no pain at this point – I could just feel every tiny part of baby's face slowly emerging, first the eyebrows, then the nose and finally the mouth and chin. I was smiling to myself while leaning against the side of the pool at this point, not only because it was such a remarkable feeling, but because I knew it was only a matter of moments before our baby would be here. Finally, with just two more pushes (only fifty minutes after having my waters broken) our baby arrived calmly, gently and safely in the water and I lifted her slowly up onto my chest. This was the point at which we discovered we had a little girl, and Ben and I just burst into tears of happiness. Our two-year-old little boy Noah had been right with his prediction throughout my entire pregnancy: he had a new little sister.

I can honestly say that giving birth to our beautiful daughter was the most amazing, positive and rewarding experience of my life — one that I thought, at one point, would never be possible until I discovered hypnobirthing. I truly believe that, without it, my daughter's birth would have been quite different.

10

Go gentle: opting for a natural caesarean

I think it's safe to say that the majority of people who come to a hypnobirthing class are not *planning* on having a caesarean – although, if you are, that's great too and this chapter is for you! But, if you're not planning one, I would stress it's important to have an open mind and be prepared. There are so many variables in pregnancy, labour and birth, which could mean that a caesarean becomes the best option for you and your baby. I have said it numerous times, but, despite perhaps having to navigate a change in your birth plan, it really is possible to have a positive, empowering and magical experience – however you welcome your baby into the world. In this chapter I will talk you through how you can make a caesarean birth the best birth possible for you.

Different types of caesarean

Firstly, it's important to acknowledge that there are different types of caesarean and to differentiate between them. There are, in fact, three types of caesarean, but the chances are that you've only ever heard of two: emergency and planned (also known as an elective caesarean). The third type of caesarean is an 'unplanned caesarean' and, despite the term not being used so frequently, it is actually the most common type of caesarean. The second most common is a 'planned caesarean' and the least common type is an 'emergency caesarean', which really is very rare.

However, I'm going to bet you've heard the phrase 'emergency caesarean' quite a bit and therefore have been led to believe it's a fairly common procedure. Perhaps you have friends who have said they have had an 'emergency caesarean'.

A *true* emergency caesarean is where the parent is put to sleep under a general anaesthetic and the birth partner is asked to leave the room. The aim is to deliver the baby as soon as possible. In this scenario somebody's life is at risk (parent and/or baby) and therefore the procedure is life-saving. But please don't worry, this really is very rare.

On reflection, knowing what you do now, I would guess that many of the stories you've heard described as emergencies actually fall into the unplanned caesarean category, where the person giving birth was awake and their birth partner was present. They were unplanned because the person went into labour planning a vaginal birth. However, things changed over the course of the labour meaning that they felt or agreed that a caesaean birth was the best option. It may well have felt like an emergency if things changed quickly, and especially if the parent wasn't informed and didn't understand what was happening at the time. Perhaps they felt scared and pressured into making a quick decision, which then increased their sense of panic. All of these factors could leave someone feeling the situation was an emergency. Or perhaps staff at the hospital referred to it as an emergency caesarean, or perhaps that was the phrase the parent was familiar with, because, as you know, 'unplanned caesarean' is not a commonly used phrase.

Whatever the reason, and certainly nobody is actively trying to fool or mislead you, it's likely that most of the people you know who have said they had emergency caesareans, actually had unplanned caesareans. This should offer you some reassurance that true emergencies are, thankfully, few and far between.

However, overall (all types combined), caesareans in the UK are a relatively common procedure; around 25 per cent of people will give birth by caesarean section each year. This figure includes unplanned, planned and emergencies. In some hospitals this percentage can be much higher.

Reassuringly, though, if you're deemed to be 'low-risk', that is, if you have no known or pre-existing medical conditions, and are enjoying a straightforward, uncomplicated pregnancy, then the likelihood of requiring a caesarean falls dramatically. For example, if you fall within this 'low-risk' category and have planned a home birth, the chance of ending up giving birth by caesarean falls to *less* than 3 per cent. Similarly, if you're 'low-risk' and giving birth at a freestanding birth centre, the chance of you having a caesarean is 3.5 per cent. At an attached birth centre or alongside midwifery unit (a midwife-led birth centre or ward on the grounds of a hospital), it's 4.4 per cent. Interestingly (or rather shockingly), if you're the same 'low-risk' person with no known medical conditions enjoying an uncomplicated pregnancy but opt to give birth on a labour ward, then the chance of giving birth by caesarean increases to over 11 per cent.[18] Meaning, statistically, you're approximately *four times* more likely to have a caesarean *just* by being on a labour ward compared to at home, even when nothing else changes and you have no known risk factors. This goes to show what an important decision choosing *where* to give birth really is: never underestimate the impact of the environment!

Of course, if you *do* have identified risk factors or known medical issues, or have experienced complications in your pregnancy, then giving birth on a labour ward could be the right and indeed *best* place for you. If you need consultant care then you need to be on a labour ward, because at home and in birth centres your care will be midwife-led. For some people, being on the labour ward *will* be the safest place for them and their baby. Remember, it's all about being informed and making choices that are right for you and your baby.

Now there may be some of you reading this who are planning a caesarean birth and I want you to know that everything I'm about to discuss is 100 per cent relevant for you. The fact you have time to plan how you want your caesarean to happen is a real bonus. After reading this chapter you should be able to draw up your own set of comprehensive birth preferences and have the opportunity to discuss your wishes with those providing your care in advance of the big day.

However, based on the law of probability, I'm going to guess that the majority of you reading this chapter aren't planning a caesarean birth. But please do remember what I said at the outset: there is a time and a place for everything. If, in the course of your pregnancy or indeed your birth, it becomes apparent that a caesarean might be the best option for you and your baby, and you opt to bring your baby into the world in this way, then you're going to want to know how to make that a positive experience.

The good news – and there's always potential for good news with a little bit of positive reframing – is that a caesarean birth can not only be a positive experience but an incredible, magical, calm and immensely empowering one. It can be *everything* you want, bar your baby coming out of your vagina. Remember I told you that the mechanics of how birth happens matter little? This is the sort of scenario I was referring to! Perhaps your baby won't be born in the exact way you imagine, but the feelings you experience (and remember those are what matter most) can be all you'd hoped for.

You're probably wondering: How can this be? If we were to

plot births on a spectrum, a caesarean birth is probably the most medicalised birth possible. Well, let me tell you about 'gentle' or 'natural' caesareans.

'Gentle' or 'natural' caesareans

A gentle or natural caesarean (the words are used interchangeably) is where as many elements as possible of vaginal birth are replicated in theatre. The most profound difference between a traditional caesarean and a natural one is that when the surgeon makes the incision, instead of pulling apart the muscles of the uterus and lifting the baby quickly out, the surgeon gently frees the baby's head through the incision and then leaves the baby to slowly make their way out, just as they would if they were descending down the birth canal and being born vaginally. This can take a few minutes, although if the surgeon frees the baby's shoulders it can be much quicker. Parents can watch their baby enter the world by choosing to have a transparent screen or no screen at all.

This method offers many benefits for both the birthing parent and their baby. For one, healing and recovery in the postnatal period is quicker as the procedure is more gentle. Secondly, the birth is slower, calmer and less alarming for baby, and they are gently squeezed as they are born just as they would be if they were born vaginally, helping them to clear the fluid from their lungs. Babies born via caesarean are statistically more likely to have respiratory issues at birth and it's believed this could be down to the fact they have bypassed the vaginal exit where they would have been slowly and gently squished, clearing their lungs.

The next key difference is that after baby is born they are lifted straight up and placed on their parent's chest and the cord is left intact. This is recommended best practice with vaginal birth, but with a traditional caesarean, the cord is usually cut quickly and the baby is taken away, cleaned up, checked over and weighed, and their paperwork is completed before being returned already wrapped up. If both parent and baby are well, there is no reason at all why they cannot enjoy immediate skin-to-skin in theatre. If it's not possible for the birthing parent to have baby on *their* chest, then baby can have immediate skin-to-skin with the birth partner. To facilitate this skin-to-skin after birth, you can request that any monitoring devices are not placed on your chest, leaving it clear to receive your baby. You can also have your gown kept loose so that it can be pulled down for easy access after birth.

The benefits of skin-to-skin and delayed cord clamping are numerous but include, for the parent: better bonding, reducing the risk of postnatal depression, reducing blood loss after birth and increasing the success rate of breastfeeding. Benefits for baby include: hearing their parent's heartbeat, which is calming and reassuring, feeling more settled after birth, early bonding, establishing breastfeeding, receiving all of their blood and not being short-changed (this alone is believed to offer lifelong benefits).

Many of these elements are considered the norm (and, indeed, recommended best practice) when it comes to vaginal birth, but are sadly still not routine when it comes to caesarean birth, despite the fact that the practices mentioned above offer the *same* benefits for babies born in theatre as they do for babies born at home or in a birth pool. It could even be argued that, for babies born by caesarean, the benefits of the above-mentioned practices are even more significant. Which is why it's so important to know your options, understand the benefits and risks of each option, and feel empowered enough to request (demand if necessary!) the birth you want for yourself and your baby.

Thankfully, increasing numbers of hospitals are offering gentle or natural caesareans, so it could be the case that you'll be offered these things before even having to ask. But if your hospital doesn't explicitly offer you a gentle or natural caesarean option, or doesn't label it as such, you can always ask for all that I've outlined above and those providing your care have a duty to respect your wishes. They can offer their advice and explain the guidelines, but ultimately they need to respect and honour your preferences – not that I anticipate you coming up against any resistance, because everything you are asking for is evidence-based with recognised benefits. In the unlikely event, however, that you did encounter someone who made you feel your preferences were not important, or that what you requested was 'not the way it's done here', I want you to know that you can say: 'I hear you, but this is the way it's happening today.' Because, guess what? *Your* body, *your* baby, *your* birth and *your* choice.

If a caesarean is on the cards, I urge you to go away and do a little more research on gentle and natural caesareans so you can better understand the full scope of the options available to you and the benefits. Knowledge is power after all! And remember, it's never too late to change hospitals either. If there's one nearby which specialises in gentle or natural caesareans, but it's not your local one, you might consider switching if a caesarean is likely or planned.

BIRTH STORY

Planned, scheduled 'natural' caesarean
birth – Kate, a second-time parent

I had a difficult birth with my first baby: my waters broke at home and then nothing. After two failed inductions and three days in labour I ended up having a very rushed and highly stressful unplanned C-section. I was beyond desperate to not have this happen with my next baby. It was and, still is, the worst experience of my life. I was adamant I was not having another C-section.

I'd had appointments with my consultant throughout this pregnancy and we both agreed I would give birth vaginally. However, at my thirty-six-week appointment I was measuring very big and after a scan I found out I had gestational diabetes. Due to my previous history and added stress of the diabetes it was decided that I was to have an elective C-section at thirty-nine weeks.

I couldn't believe it. I felt like a failure all over again. I had really wanted to have this baby vaginally, but it wasn't to be. I decided to throw myself into hypnobirthing and use it to my advantage. I wanted to wipe away all the bad memories of the previous experience and treat this as a whole new beginning.

On the big day, it was such a surreal feeling waking up and knowing our baby was to be born today. We went off to hospital and I was second in on the list – a little daunting as it meant more time to think about what was about to happen, but also allowed time to mentally prepare. Adam and I filled this time making a 'birth playlist' I felt I could relax to in the moment. At my pre-op, I asked the surgeon to do a 'natural C-section' – a huge thing for me due to the bad memories of the previous op and being so bloody squeamish. But I was determined this was to be as natural as possible, and so the lights were dimmed and the theatre team were quiet.

All was going well until I started to panic and go into shock. Adam was absolutely fantastic in calming me down, stroking my arm and doing the breathing techniques, in for four, out for *eight to relax me. I listened to my playlist and closed my eyes, constantly breathing; it worked – I relaxed and, before I knew it, the team asked if I was ready for the curtain to be brought down.*

We watched our baby being born and it was such a relaxed and calm experience – it was truly beautiful. We asked for delayed cord cutting and I had my baby placed on my chest for skin-to-skin. It was and always will be one of the best experiences of my life. They stayed there for the duration of the operation, only coming off for Adam to cut their cord, and went on to feed straight away whilst we were still in theatre. The recovery physically was still difficult but mentally I felt in such a better place.

I can't believe that two similar situations can end up being so different and I have Siobhan's course to thank for enabling me to experience something so special and for turning my worst experience into one of my best experiences. I have completely come to terms with my labours and what I achieved in having both my children. How lucky we are to have them. Birth is amazing no matter how it happens.

Caesarean birth preferences

Even if a caesarean isn't on the cards, I still recommend undertaking a little inquisitive research and outlining your preferences on your birth preferences document, in case a caesarean should become necessary. I have had three babies, all vaginally, but have always included my preferences for a caesarean. Remember, there's a time and place for everything, including intervention. Pregnancy and birth can be unpredictable and it would be naive of us to assume none of us will ever need any assistance. So, for that reason I have always included my preferences for a caesarean on my main birth preferences document, even though I have always planned for a vaginal birth.

The likelihood is that you won't need to use them, but if you do then you have them ready. Better that than be in a situation where you've made the decision to go to theatre for an unplanned caesarean and you're desperately trying to think back to what you read in some book (this one!) months before. That doesn't bode well for a calm and relaxed birth experience. So, take the time now to give it some thought, note down your preferences and then go forth focusing on the vaginal birth you want (if indeed, that is what you want!).

If you're planning a caesarean then the focus of your birth preferences document will obviously be on how you wish the caesarean to be done. You might, however, consider including a small paragraph on what you wish to happen should you end up having an unplanned vaginal birth. Because, like I said, pregnancy and birth can be unpredictable!

Using your hypnobirthing techniques in theatre

In addition to the elements that form part of a gentle or natural caesarean, you also have other options in theatre that are worth giving some consideration to and including in your birth preferences document. For example, you might like to give some thought to the environment. When it comes to creating the right setting for birth, we have established that a dark, quiet, private space in which you feel safe is optimum. Consider how you might be able to create that space in theatre using your five senses checklist.

You can request that the lights be turned off or down, and that the surgeon works with a spotlight so that they can see what they are doing, leaving the rest of the room in darkness.

You could bring in your battery-operated tea lights and place them around so they are in your sight line. You can have your choice of music playing in theatre. You can use an essential oil roller ball if this aids your relaxation and you can bring in your own pillow or blanket. Your birth partner will be there, by your side and on your side, and you can use all of your relaxation tools and hypnobirthing techniques in order to remain calm, so that you are able to meet your baby feeling relaxed and happy, confident and capable. Just because you aren't experiencing surges in theatre doesn't mean that your up breathing will no longer be of use. Remember, it is essentially a calming breath and can be used in *all* situations in life where you feel anxious or overwhelmed. And it's quite natural to feel this way when heading to theatre for what could be your very first major operation. So, use your up breathing to calm you, the arm stroking to help you relax and whatever else you have to hand in your toolbox. It's good to know that when it comes to birth, there is no situation where being calm and relaxed won't help. Your tools can be used for *all* births and will make your birth better.

Lastly, although you won't need oxytocin to help you dilate in theatre, remember that oxytocin is responsible for more than just surges: it aids bonding by helping to establish breastfeeding, it reduces the risk of postnatal depression, and it helps the uterus to contract after birth, thus reducing blood loss. So, the more oxytocin you have in your body at birth (however the birth happens), the better. All of your relaxation tools will get your natural oxytocin flowing, so embrace them in theatre, just as you would anywhere else.

Remember, just as with vaginal birth, this is *your* body, *your* baby, *your* birth and most importantly *your* choice! And even if you feel your choices are becoming more limited, it's important to know that you still always have choices about how you bring your baby into this world. I have heard people say that they felt disappointed after giving birth by caesarean, but if it's a choice *you* made because it was the *best option* for you and your baby, then really that's something to be proud of. Often a little positive reframing is helpful in these situations. We are lucky to have the option of caesarean available to us, and when it's needed we can embrace it. After all, we all want to birth our babies safely and in the best way possible on the day, and sometimes that will be by caesarean. If you ever feel unsure about what course of action to take, remember you can always rely on the B.R.A.I.N. framework to ensure you're making informed decisions that feel right for you and your baby, and then navigate your birth – however it turns out – feeling calm, relaxed and confident by using all of your hypnobirthing toolkit. *You've got this!*

Having taught so many people hypnobirthing over the past few years, I can recall many positive caesarean birth stories and truly believe that birth in theatre can be a hugely positive and empowering experience, enabling you to bring your baby into the world feeling calm, confident and strong, just as you hoped.

BIRTH STORY

Unplanned caesarean – Natalie, first-time parent

I had a few twinges Saturday afternoon, so drank my raspberry leaf tea, carried around a tissue with clary sage and got the take-away menu out to choose a Saturday night curry! By the time we had finished our curry, we knew baby was on the way and had started timing contractions.

We set up our 'nest' at home and, as I was unable to sleep through or in between the surges, we lit candles, watched

Friends on TV, and had lots of cuddles and massage, and I kept focused on the up breathing and affirmations.

By 3am we headed to the MLU and the team there were fab. I said I was happy to be checked, and they confirmed I was 4cm dilated, suggesting a bath while they finished cleaning/preparing the pool delivery room for us.

I happily got in the bath and it felt amazing. My boyfriend helped me maintain up breathing and an hour later I was feeling in the zone. My boyfriend then heard a pop and looked into the bath. My waters had broken and it was clear that there was meconium in the water with me. Two midwives came to help and supported me as I stood up and out onto a pad.

I was taken to the labour ward and advised that there was a considerable amount of meconium (and of a certain consistency), which gave them cause for concern and they wanted to monitor baby.

We knew this would mean a certain amount of restriction, but we talked it through together, used our B.R.A.I.N. and agreed. We also talked openly with the team and asked them to support us in continuing towards a vaginal birth (even though we knew water birth was now out of the question).

The team was great, talked us through our options and we 'laboured on'. I started using gas and air and got completely in the zone – I looked at and talked to only my boyfriend for about four hours while I followed his lead on the up breathing, lots of eye contact and reassurance. It was a bonding experience between the two of us that I will cherish forever; I've never felt such incredible closeness and connection with another person.

The team praised me throughout for staying calm and

several people made reference to a very low resting heart rate – apparently I stayed below 60bpm and they couldn't believe it.

Other than the bond with my boyfriend, I don't have many memories from this stage – it felt a little 'other worldly' and really quite magic! After four hours we had progressed to 6cm but then baby's heart rate started dipping. We were shown the charts and talked through our options. We used our B.R.A.I.N. and decided to go to theatre for a C-section.

I used the head and face relaxation recording, as well as up breathing, to keep focused and stay calm, and baby was with us twenty minutes later. There was lots of skin-to-skin time with us, and breastfeeding within thirty minutes.

So, our labour and delivery were not at all as we had imagined, but we felt informed and consulted throughout the journey, we stayed calm and collected and worked together as a couple and as a team with the hospital staff . . . and ultimately came away with what had always been our goal – a happy, healthy baby.

11

The big day (or night)

So you've got the toolkit, you've put in the hours and you're primed and ready to go! But what happens when everything kicks off for real? When should you travel to the birth centre or hospital, or make the call if having a home birth? When should you start with the up breathing? When should you stop? When should your birth partner deploy the arm stroking or light-touch massage? Should you hold out for the pool? Who's going to make the birthing space look and smell like a spa?

If you're reading this feeling like your brain is full of information and you're worried that you will forget it all once labour starts: *Do. Not. Fear.* In this chapter, I'm going to explain what to do when, and I promise it really is all quite logical and straightforward.

The good news is that if you're the one who is currently growing the baby, you're doing the bulk of the work right now, and, sure, you have to birth the baby too, but when it comes to the birth there's only one thing you need to focus on – and that's breathing. That's it! Breathing. For the majority of the time, whenever you feel a surge coming on, inhale through your nose for a count of four, feeling your chest expand, then slowly exhale through your mouth for a count of eight, feeling all tension release as everything softens and relaxes. And just do that on repeat. Easy peasy! You shouldn't have to worry about doing anything else or indeed worry about *anything* at all! The more relaxed you are, the more comfortable everything will feel and the more efficient your surges will be – making birth quicker, easier and more straightforward, which, after all, is the aim of the game!

This is why you need a birth partner or two to support you: so you can focus on relaxation and they can take care of the lengthy 'to-do' list. If you don't yet have a birth partner in place I'd really recommend trying to get one on board. Obviously, I can't know every individual's situation and I don't wish to make assumptions, but if you haven't got a partner or family member to support you, then consider asking a friend or looking into doula schemes local to you. It is possible to get a volunteer doula, or even an NHS-employed doula, in different parts of the country. More information can be found on the Doula UK website (see Resources on page 231). No one should have to go into birth alone and there are projects in place to support those who most need it.

So there really is no need to feel overwhelmed by the tasks – you have got a single focus: breathing, the happy side effect of which is relaxation. It's near impossible to panic if you remain committed to the up-breathing technique.

Birth partners, however ... you have quite the list to complete, which is why the job you're doing is both significant in size and importance. You are an integral part of the birthing team, charged with bringing a new human into the world. No pressure now! Remember how I told you that no more is the birth partner a spare part, a third wheel, or whatever other analogy is commonly used, but an essential and imperative cog in the system? If it takes two to make a baby, it takes a team to birth a baby and, indeed, some would say a whole village to raise one.

Teamwork really does make the dream work! Or at the very least, makes it a lot easier.

This is why, if you're pregnant, you need to choose your birth partner (or partners) wisely. The job requirements include the ability to multitask, remain calm under pressure, and have the confidence to advocate for you and, if necessary, challenge authority. Birth partners, if you're reading this, know that you are well capable of rising to the job! Do not doubt yourself: you have got this! You are a strong and capable human. (This is not the first time the thought has crossed my mind that I ought to produce some confidence-boosting affirmations for birth partners as well as for those who are pregnant!)

To help make sense of everything that has been covered thus far, I'm going to go through the stages of labour that we have discussed previously, in chronological order from early labour through to the third and final stage, outlining exactly what you might be doing at each stage and where you might be. I'll also give you a clear action list so that everyone knows what they're meant to be doing. By breaking it down in this way, I hope it will feel less overwhelming.

Early labour

During early labour you're most likely to be at home, even if you plan on giving birth at a birth centre or hospital. If you travel into a birth centre or hospital whilst still in early labour you're very likely to be sent home. This can feel frustrating and disappointing and disrupts the progression of labour, not to mention that travelling back and forth is annoying and a waste of your time. For all these reasons, settle down at home and wait until things are well established before going anywhere.

Early labour can be a really wonderful time because the surges will be mild and irregular, giving you plenty of time to practise all your lovely relaxation exercises. Now is the time to get the oxytocin flowing, because, as you know, oxytocin is the magic that fuels the surges and will help get things more established. Being relaxed is key to producing oxytocin, so anything and everything that helps you to relax is good to do now!

Endorphins are also very helpful in birth, given that they are your body's natural pain relief. Unlike other hormones, endorphins hang around in the body for some time, so producing a good bank of them now in early labour is only a good thing and will hopefully see you through when things become more powerful.

You can get the endorphins flowing through exercise and, because your body is essentially working out in labour – the uterus muscles will be working hard – this will be happening anyway. However, light-touch massage and a TENS machine are effective in boosting your production of endorphins. Both work in a similar way by stimulating the nerves in the spine.

With regard to how active you should or shouldn't be, the feedback is mixed. I always advocate listening to your body and, of course, the time of day (or night) also influences matters. If it's the middle of the night (as is often the case), then try and sleep if you can. It's quite possible that things will build whilst you are resting, but you will definitely be woken when the surges become more powerful – there's no fear of you sleeping through and missing the main event! Likewise, going to sleep won't bring things to a halt if it's the real thing. It's always better to go into labour and birth on the back of a good night's sleep, rather than set off from the starter blocks in the disadvantaged position of having missed out. In fact, when it comes to pregnancy, birth and parenting, a good rule of thumb is: never miss an opportunity to sleep. Once your baby is here you will come to appreciate every moment of sleep. Sleep is so important for your well-being.

Saying that, if you can't sleep, try to at least rest. I know I've talked about being in a good U.F.O. position to speed things up – being upright with gravity on your side means baby's head will weigh down on the cervix, helping to speed up dilation – but if it's the middle of the night and you're tired (as is normal), then lying on your left-hand side and resting is no bad thing. You may find in early labour that you're able to drift in and out of sleep in this position. Maybe play a guided relaxation MP3, or your positive affirmations, and allow your subconscious to absorb these positive messages as you rest in preparation.

If it's the daytime and you feel wide awake, then, again, listen to your body. There's no point lying down and trying to sleep if you don't feel at all sleepy! It's true that being upright will help get things going and speed up progress. Gravity combined with the weight of baby's head is a powerful combination. If you're at home, perhaps you could use a birth ball, if you have one, or stand up and lean over a counter or sink to support yourself. Or even a table. You might find it comfortable to kneel and hug the birth ball or lean over the side of the sofa. Maybe you might fancy going for a walk and getting some fresh air. Whatever feels right for *you* – do that. Remember, the most important thing is to be relaxed so that your body can do its amazing, miraculous thing.

Early labour can be variable from person to person, and even from one person's birth to the next. There are so many factors that can affect how early labour goes. It's unpredictable, which can be frustrating. We all want to know 'Is this it?' and whether it's your first baby or fourth, you're still going to be asking yourself this question in early labour – because there is no real way of ever knowing if this really is it. Sometimes early labour can build in momentum and it becomes obvious that this really is *it*, but at other times early labour can tail off – everything grinds to a halt and it becomes obvious that this is *not* it. It's common for early labour to be a bit stop-start.

For some people early labour can last many days, with surges picking up and then petering out; for others it can last less than an hour – or even be under fifteen minutes if labour becomes established very quickly. Both scenarios have pros and cons. A labour that establishes itself very quickly can be quite intense from the offset with no gradual build-up, giving you less time to get your space sorted and practise relaxation exercises. A speedy labour can feel like a bit of a whirlwind, so, much as everyone dreams of a fast labour, there are definitely pros to a slower build-up. If you have a longer early labour, try your best to relax and enjoy it. This is a great opportunity to practise your relaxation, knowing that your body is doing its thing. Place your trust in your body and your baby, and focus on the fact that you will be meeting your baby soon. Every surge is doing something – none is wasted. This *can* be a very calm, gentle and magical time.

At some point, however, the surges will build in three ways: frequency, duration and intensity. You need all three elements to come together for labour to be considered established. You want the surges to be coming approximately three in ten, which, remember, means three surges in each ten-minute period, and for that pattern to be well established – the 'frequency' element. You also want each surge to last between forty-five seconds and a minute – that's the 'duration' element. Finally, you want the surges to be nice and strong! There's no point in having lots of mild surges for hours and hours that are not very effective. You want strong, effective surges, so embrace them as they grow in power – this is the 'intensity' element. I've actually created an app to help you time your surges (you'll find it listed in the resources section at the back of this book). It also guides you through your breathing and helps you to relax between surges.

Using the app makes it easy to keep track of what's going on over a period of time. But, of course, the good old-fashioned method of pen and paper, together with a clock or watch, works as well.

Once you've reached that magic 3/10/45, then it's time to make the journey into the birth centre or hospital, or to call the midwife out to you if having a home birth. You can now consider yourself to be in established or active labour, or the first stage (different names all meaning the same thing). This is where the official timing of labour begins. Everything that has gone before this point is considered early labour and doesn't contribute towards the official length of labour.

Hospitals or birth centres consider you to be in established labour once you are 4cm dilated, but, given that you're likely to be at home during early labour, it's obviously not possible to gauge how many centimetres dilated you are yourself. Instead, focus on the frequency, duration and intensity of the surges. Lots of people who have had babies previously will look you in the eye and say: 'You just *know*', which always sounds very unhelpful. (But how will I know?) However, it's true. You *will* know. Even if this is your first experience of birth and you've never done this before; you *will* know. Trust your body and your baby (and your instincts) – your body and baby both know what they are doing.

In summary, here are some things you could do during the early stage of labour:

- Go for a walk in nature
- Eat some food
- Stay hydrated
- Have a lie-down
- Have a bath
- Watch a funny or happy movie
- Listen to an enjoyable podcast

- Listen to your positive affirmations
- Listen to a guided relaxation MP3
- Lower the lights, use essential oils, play relaxing or happy music
- Have a cuddle
- Light-touch massage
- Use a TENS machine
- Practise your guided relaxation exercises with your birth partner
- Bounce on a birth ball
- Have a shower
- Arm stroking
- Up breathing

Established labour

You're now in proper established labour. This is the real deal. You've travelled into the hospital or birth centre, or your midwife has come out to you. You're probably expecting me to tell you that this is where it gets difficult? Wrong! This is where it gets easy – in a way!

You now have a single focus. You are in the right place (that *you* have chosen), you are being supported by your birth partner (they are not just by your side but *on* your side), your baby is on its way (whoop!) and your job now is simply to relax. Your focus will become more channelled now and the only thing you need to remember to do is breathe: in for four, out for eight, four times over, rest and repeat.

It sounds simple – and it really is! Breathing is now your sole focus; use the up-breathing technique through each surge and relax in between. Every time you feel a surge come on (which you can expect to happen approximately three times in every ten-minute period) simply close your eyes, inhale through your nose, feel your chest expand before exhaling slowly through your mouth, and feel all tension release as you become more deeply relaxed. Perhaps you will have your birth partner count for you to coach you through each one and keep you grounded and focused. Perhaps you will rely on the powerful visualis-ations that you've been practising – visualising, for example, a hot air balloon inflating and filling up with air as you inhale and then, as you exhale, seeing the balloon gracefully glide up and up and away. There's no right or wrong way; whichever method works best for you is great.

And, reassuringly, you know that you only have to commit to that breathing pattern for four cycles, which is approximately forty-eight seconds, by which time the surge will have either passed entirely or certainly be on the release; you know that when you open your eyes you will be one step closer to meeting your baby.

Also, know that it doesn't get 'harder' from this point. Something that people often ask me is, once the surges feel really strong and powerful, how will they cope if they get even stronger? The good news is that, generally, once that pattern is established – 3/10/45 – it stays that way. The surges don't become more frequent, last for longer or become stronger. You might start to feel more tired, as with any workout, but the pattern tends to stay the same. Some people report that right near the very end the surges feel more intense and come a little faster, but that is usually when they are mere moments from meeting their baby.

This stage really has a lot more to do with your mental, rather than physical strength: it's about releasing any worries you might be holding on to, focusing on positive thoughts, allowing your body to relax and open each time you feel a surge come on, and having the strength of mind to commit to that breath and see it all the way through. It can feel intense at the peak, but remember, you can do *anything* for sixty seconds!

In between surges, you might like to exchange some words with your birth partner, move to a more comfortable position, have some sips of a drink or even a little snack. The main thing is to ensure that you're returning to 'green' after each surge – that state of complete relaxation in mind and body.

And that really is it! You may well be doing this for several hours, but soon enough it will be time to meet the baby that you've been waiting to hold for what probably feels like a lifetime.

Birth partners, on the other hand, I'm not going to lie, you are going to be kept busy!

Whether on arrival at the birth centre or hospital, or if staying at home, the first thing birth partners need to do is to set the scene. Think back to the five senses: sight, sound, smell, taste, touch. Aim to address each one as though you are working through a five-point checklist. Are each of the five senses being met with something that brings comfort and aids relaxation? If not, then change that thing.

You will probably adjust the lighting first as this makes the most profound difference to a space. The dimmer and darker the better. You might be arranging battery-operated tea lights around the room or lighting candles at home. You might have a string of fairy lights to put up. Then there's sound and smell. Perhaps you have a playlist to play or positive affirmations, or a familiar guided relaxation. Then maybe you're spritzing the room with a scented room spray. You're also making sure that the person giving birth feels comfortable and supported, that they are wearing comfy clothes with which they have positive associations, that they feel relaxed and at ease, and, finally, that you're offering them drinks and snacks so that they remain hydrated and energised.

This might seem like a lot but if you work through the five senses as a checklist it can be done in a few moments after arrival at a birth centre or hospital. And if you're at home there's no need to wait until things are established to create a happy, tranquil space conducive for relaxation.

Ideally this is the first job the birth partner does, because, as I've said before, the surroundings have such a huge impact on how labour pans out. By packing a few choice items in advance you have the power to change a setting in a matter of minutes. For example, a brightly lit, sterile, hospital room can be quickly transformed into a romantic and intimate candlelit space that smells of essential oils and sounds like a spa, where there's the option to rest on a cosy blanket and tuck into treats. Very swiftly it becomes a blissful place where you *want* to be, a place where you *enjoy* being and a space in which you can relax, let go and birth a baby.

Next up, after setting the scene, your job (birth partners!) is primarily to provide support through the surges. This means being physically there with the person giving birth, by their side, but also letting them know you are on their side and will advocate for them if necessary and protect the space. If they know this, and have a birth partner they can trust, they can allow themself to be vulnerable and relax further. Someone who is anxious about who will advocate for them, who is worrying about the environment and the job list and who will do what, will struggle to fully let go and relax. So be the kind of birth partner that creates an environment which enables the parent giving birth to feel safe; let them know you have their back.

From this point on, you're focusing on supporting and coaching the parent giving birth through their surges. You may count slowly and methodically to help them pace their breathing, or they may prefer for there to be silence and to rely on their own visualisations. Even in silence, by physically being there and being present they will feel safer and be able to relax further.

In between surges your job is to help the parent who is giving birth to return to that 'green' state where they are completely relaxed. You have lots of tools you can use to achieve this. For example, light-touch massage or arm stroking. Reassuring words can work wonders here, as well as simple actions such as resting your hands on their shoulders and encouraging them to let them drop and relax. You also have the arm-dropping technique to encourage the release of any tension they might be holding onto in their body.

Between surges is also the time to offer drinks and perhaps even snacks. It's very important to stay hydrated during labour and they may well forget to ask for a drink because they are so focused and preoccupied. So be sure to have one to hand and be offering it regularly.

You might have other items packed in the birth bag that you can use to help them relax, and between surges is the time to use them. Massage oil for example. Or a cool flannel to hold against their forehead or neck. Perhaps they have a refreshing face spray or head massager. You can use any and all of these tools as long as they are aiding relaxation.

Don't forget about the environment as labour progresses – perhaps you will need to re-spritz the room if using a room spray for scent or reapply essential oils if using a rollerball. Perhaps you will need to change the music or play some positive affirmations or a favourite guided relaxation at points.

Then, if necessary, birth partners, you will need to be prepared to advocate and ensure their wishes are respected. You should have a copy (or a few copies) of their birth preferences document for reference. Make sure you request that those providing the care have a read of the document and, if there's a shift change, that any new midwife or doctor also has a copy to read. You can also refer to the document to remind yourself what their wishes are so that you're in a good position to quickly respond if you feel they are not being followed.

Finally, if things start to change, birth partners, you will need to engage your B.R.A.I.N. and ask those five important questions:

1. What are the Benefits?
2. What are the Risks?
3. Are there any Alternatives?
4. What does my Instinct say?
5. What happens if we do Nothing for X amount of time?

You can't make any decisions on anyone else's behalf, but you can help them make an informed decision by asking the right questions and gathering all the necessary information to enable them to make an *informed* choice. You might feel like the go-between, but you're playing an important role by doing so – empowering the parent who is giving birth to make the right choice for them and baby!

You may never need to use your B.R.A.I.N., and hopefully everything will unfold in a straightforward way with no need to deviate from the birth preferences outlined. However, if something does arise, you'll have the framework and tools to deal with it calmly and confidently, working like a team to bring baby into the world calmly and in the best way possible.

I should also mention that if you're planning a home birth, birth partners you'll also have the job of inflating and filling the birth pool (if you have one). This can be a job in itself and I would thoroughly recommend doing a practice run first (ensure you have a sterile, unopened liner kept aside for the real day if doing so!). You want to know for sure in advance that the hose adaptor fits the tap to avoid any last-minute dashes to a hardware store during the labour – which, in case it needs clarifying, is definitely *not* going to aid anyone's relaxation!

If you're planning a birth-centre or hospital birth you don't have to worry about the pool – that will be sorted by the midwives if you have requested to use one, and one is available. The downside here is that you now have the added job of arranging the transfer in. You might be driving and therefore needing to make a plan regarding parking and potentially dropping the pregnant parent at the entrance beforehand. Alternatively, perhaps you have a friend or family member who can drive you in and drop you at the entrance together, or you might take a taxi to avoid having to find a parking space. Whatever you choose to do, I would recommend making a plan for your journey in advance so it's not something you have to stress about on the day. Minimal stress, maximum relaxation – that's what we're aiming for here!

So, to summarise, these are the things someone might do, or benefit from doing, during the first stage of labour, and which you can assist with:

- Up breathing through the surges
- Relaxing in between surges
- Regular sips of a drink
- Light snacks
- Remembering U.F.O. – assuming an upright, forward and open position

Birth partners, here are some of the things you might be doing:

- Organising the transfer to the birth centre or hospital, or arranging a midwife to come out
- If at home, potentially inflating and filling the pool

- Setting the scene using the five senses checklist
- Providing support through the surges by counting
- Using your toolkit to help the parent giving birth to relax and return to 'green' in between the surges
- Light-touch massage
- Arm stroking
- Arm drop
- Guided relaxations
- Positive affirmations and words of reassurance and encouragement
- Offering drinks frequently and snacks if required
- Ensuring everyone has a copy of the birth preferences document
- Ensuring the birth preferences are respected and advocating if necessary
- Maintaining the environment/protecting the space
- Acting as the gatekeeper to the room so communication goes through you
- Using your B.R.A.I.N. if necessary to equip the parent giving birth with the information they need to make an informed decision
- Encouraging the person birthing to use a U.F.O. position

The final stretch

Now that your body has started pushing down, you know you have entered the second stage of labour. You'll know because you can feel it – a powerful, involuntary pushing sensation from within that you wouldn't be able to stop, even if you wanted to!

During this second stage, again, you have little to do but focus on your breathing and remain relaxed. At this stage you will be using your down-breathing technique: take a big, quick breath in through the nose to fill the lungs, then exhale through your mouth with focus and intent, channelling your breath down through your body and feeling your uterus muscles responding.

You do not need to push, although your muscles will be pushing powerfully. Rather, you should concentrate on breathing through the powerful surges in a focused way, essentially breathing your baby out. This might sound impossible to some, especially as we only ever see people on the TV being coached to push (often forcefully), but it really is possible and ensures a gentle birth for your body and your baby. Take time to read some positive birth stories and you'll feel more confident that this *can* and *will* happen! Most importantly, remember to just keep on breathing!

Another helpful thing to remember at this stage, which the breathing will help with, is to remain as relaxed as possible and allow everything to soften and open on a muscular level. Sometimes opening visualisations can be helpful – for example a rosebud blossoming and opening. Visualisations can be a powerful tool for some but do nothing for others. It really is personal preference whether you choose to use visualisations or not. But, either way, if you are relaxed and allowing everything to soften and open, it will make for a quicker and easier down stage and birth.

In order to allow all your muscles to soften and relax, you need to be relaxed in your mind. Remind yourself that you've done all the hard work now and you're so close to meeting your baby. Welcome the sensation of your baby descending, knowing that you are mere moments from holding them in your arms. Allow your pelvic floor to release, your shoulders to drop, your arms to rest limp and relaxed. Focus on returning to this 'green' state between each downwards surge.

And lastly, get gravity on your side! It *will* help. Put simply, your baby will descend faster if you are upright, and each downwards surge will be more effective if the weight of baby's head is pushing down and helping everything to gently stretch and open. Gravity and the uterus muscles are a very powerful combo. As always, a good U.F.O. position will make for an easier birth and significantly reduces your risk of requiring assistance and also of experiencing a tear.

Birth partners: you'll be pleased to know you have *slightly* less to do during this active second stage of labour. The key thing for you to do now is to remain present for the person giving birth. Remember the mantra: '*by* your side and *on* your side'. Offer them encouragement as the finishing line is now firmly in sight and they could be feeling tired. The sensation they are experiencing is a new one and unlike what they have felt before. Not necessarily more intense, just a different feeling as the body takes over and begins to push and baby descends through the pelvis. You now take on the role of cheerleader! Remind the parent giving birth to focus and use their breath (just as they have practised) and to work *with* their body rather than against it. If they are holding their breath, bracing or resisting the sensation of this down stage, it will slow down progress and make it more difficult. This stage will be quicker, easier, more straightforward and more comfortable if they focus on using their down breathing. So remind them of this, if appropriate, and perhaps breathe in sync with them to help keep them on track.

In between each surge your job is the same: help them to return to the 'green state' of relaxation. Any tension that has accumulated during the surge, now is the time to encourage them to let it go. You could use the arm-stroking technique here, light-touch massage or even the arm drop. You might offer reassurance or whisper positive affirmations. Above all, you will be present and offer reassurance and encouragement. This is a very active stage; the baby is descending and being born. You are on the verge of witnessing the most miraculous and awesome thing of your entire life. Allow yourself to feel excited and pass on these positive vibes. They too will help!

Remember to offer sips of water or whatever drink it is that the person in labour wishes to have, just as you were doing previously. The muscles work more effectively and to their full potential if they are hydrated.

If the person giving birth is feeling hot and sweaty, as they may well be because their body is working to its max, perhaps use a fan, a face spray, a cool flannel, or whatever else you have packed, to help them feel refreshed and energised.

Maintain the calm, safe and intimate environment and mentally run through the five senses checklist. You shouldn't have much more to do here at this stage because everything has already been set up, but just do a little last-minute check and ensure that each of the five senses are being met with something that brings comfort and offers reassurance, helping the parent giving birth to relax their body and allow it to open. If there is anything, however small, that you believe could introduce some level of tension, seek to remove it from the space. When you're giving birth, your senses will be particularly heightened at this stage. Subconsciously you will be scanning the environment for any potential threat, so it's important that you feel safe and protected now, in order to birth your baby. Therefore, birth partners, make sure nothing threatens to disturb the feeling of peace and calm in the room.

The environment is just as important now, if not *more* so, than it was in earlier stages of labour. As you know, oxytocin is the hormone that is fuelling the surges but is *also* the hormone that helps with bonding, reduces postnatal depression, reduces blood loss and helps get breastfeeding established. The parent giving birth will want *lots* of this when they meet their baby for the first time! And an environment which enables them to relax is key, because the more relaxed they are, the more oxytocin they will produce.

Lastly encourage the parent who is giving birth to adopt a U.F.O. (upright, forward, open) position and offer some physical support if needed. A good U.F.O. position could be standing upright and leaning over something, squatting, using a birthing stool, kneeling, on all fours, etc. Think Upright and you have gravity, Forward to encourage optimum positioning, and Open to allow the body to open unrestricted and to its full potential.

To recap, during this second stage of labour the person giving birth might:

- Focus on down breathing through each surge
- Relax in between surges, aiming to return to the green state
- Use a U.F.O. position
- Have frequent sips of a drink to stay hydrated
- Benefit from a cold flannel or cooling face spray

Birth partners:

- Encourage the parent giving birth to breathe through the surges
- Perhaps breathe in sync *with* them
- Offer words of encouragement, reassurance and motivation
- Be a cheerleader – the finish line is in sight!
- Maintain the environment – refer to the five senses checklist and protect the space
- Act as a gatekeeper – all communication is to go through you to minimise any disturbance
- Use your B.R.A.I.N. if needed to gather necessary information

- Ensure the birth preferences are respected and be an advocate if required
- Encourage the person giving birth to use and potentially support them, in a good U.F.O. position
- Offer drinks frequently
- Aim to keep them cool, refreshed and comfortable
- Use positive affirmations
- Have a camera ready for the big moment (if that has been agreed)

Hello baby!

Wow wow wow! So baby is here! And now it's time for the precious Golden Hour. If all is well, parent and baby can now enjoy some skin-to-skin time without interruption, unless medically necessary. Skin-to-skin, as we have covered, offers numerous benefits for both the person who has given birth and the new baby.

During these initial few minutes after birth, if you have opted for delayed cord clamping your baby will still be attached via the umbilical cord to the placenta, which is yet to come out. The placenta will be returning baby's blood to baby during this time. The umbilical cord will be firm, blue in colour and pulsating as the blood flows through it. After a few minutes the cord will turn white and appear limp and empty. You know that the baby now has all of their blood back, and the cord can be clamped and cut.

At this point, if you are in the birth pool you would be encouraged to step out for the reasons that I've mentioned earlier: 1) It's hard to gauge blood loss in water. 2) The water will be getting cold (as will baby). 3) Midwives prefer you to birth the placenta on dry land so they can properly inspect it and ensure it's complete.

Once you're out of the pool, you might sit on a birth stool, on mats on the floor reclining onto bean bags, on a bed, on a sofa, on the toilet ... this is slightly dictated by where you are and what 'apparatus' you have available to you for use. It's worth bearing in mind that a good U.F.O. position will still be helpful, though. You are now waiting for the placenta to separate from the uterus wall and be birthed. As I've mentioned, this can take up to an hour. Whilst waiting you will ideally be enjoying some precious skin-to-skin time with your baby, with the pair of you wrapped up together in towels and blankets to keep you both warm. The time will pass very quickly.

You might consider putting your baby to your breast as any stimulation of the nipple will boost your production of oxytocin. Oxytocin will help the uterus surge and speed up the process of birthing the placenta, as well as sending a memo to your internal milk factory to let it know baby has been born and that it's time to get going. This also helps reduce blood loss by speeding up the process of the uterus contracting and shrinking back down, aids with bonding (being the happy love hormone) and reduces the risk of postnatal depression. So, if you feel you need a quick boost, putting your baby to your breast will help.

Soon enough you will feel that now-familiar involuntary pushing sensation from within, although nowhere near as intense as birthing a baby, you'll be pleased to know! And then you may have to give a little push yourself and you will feel the placenta pass through and out of your vagina.

This is known as a *physiological* third stage. 'Physiological' simply means natural and this is in reference to the fact that no drugs have been introduced to manage this third stage. The placenta has been birthed.

The placenta is a large organ that differs in size, depending on the person and the baby. Birthing the placenta is *not* like birthing a second baby, but likewise it's not just going to slip out without you noticing. You will have to actively *birth* it. I don't know why, but I imagined it would be jelly-like in texture and sort of flop out. I can confirm, having now seen many placentas, including my own, that this is not the case. It's actually quite chunky and firm.

If you were having an actively managed third stage things would be slightly different: the cord would likely be clamped and cut sooner after birth, and you would be encouraged to step out of the pool earlier (if you gave birth in one). You would be given an injection into your thigh and you would expect the placenta to follow soon after.

We have already covered the reasons why you might opt for active management over a physiological third stage, but just to reiterate, the most commons reasons are:

- Convenience – to speed the process up
- Concerns about blood loss – active management reduces the risk of postpartum haemorrhage (PPH) and is used to manage blood loss when PPH occurs
- To help with retained placenta (where the placenta doesn't separate spontaneously from the uterus wall as it should)

After this 'Golden Hour' is up, the parent who has given birth can then be examined and if any stitches are required, these can be done at this point. The baby is now weighed and examined, and the birth partner then has the opportunity to enjoy some skin-to-skin before putting the first nappy on, and possibly dressing the baby.

The birthing parent and baby are then reunited and ideally able to get into bed to enjoy some cuddles, and the famous post-birth tea-and-toast combo.

Birth partners, your job is getting easier now, you'll be pleased to hear! Key things to do at this stage include maintaining the environment – remember your five senses checklist. The reason for this is that it is still very important for the person who has given birth to produce lots of oxytocin post-birth, which they will do naturally if they are relaxed and feeling good. Keep the environment calm and peaceful to enable them to relax and enjoy these precious early moments. Your role is to protect the space from interruptions – there is no need in this first hour to make birth announcements or anything else. Keep activity to a minimum and respect this special time – it's called the Golden Hour for a reason.

As in the previous stages, ensure you are familiar with the birth preferences document and are able to advocate and ensure all wishes are respected when it comes to important things like skin-to-skin, cord clamping and cutting, and the delivery of the placenta. Be prepared to use your B.R.A.I.N., if necessary, and feed back all the information you've gathered to the parent who has given birth so they can make properly informed choices if any new recommendations are being made.

If it's not possible for baby to have immediate skin-to-skin with the parent who has just given birth, for whatever reason, be prepared to whip your top off so that the baby can enjoy skin-to-skin time with you. Hearing your heartbeat will offer baby reassurance and comfort as this has been the soundtrack to their entire life so far.

In summary, during the third stage the parent who has given birth might:

- Enjoy some lovely skin-to-skin cuddles with the baby
- Potentially offer the baby their breast or try chest feeding
- Have the cord clamped and cut

- Leave the pool if they have given birth in it
- Birth the placenta
- Remain relaxed throughout
- Feel like a superhero!

Birth partners will be:

- Protecting the space/maintaining the environment
- Ensuring birth preferences and wishes are respected
- Speaking up and advocating if necessary
- Using your B.R.A.I.N. if new recommendations are being made
- Enjoying newborn cuddles if appropriate

And then that's it! If you're in hospital or at a birth centre and all is well then you could be going home in matter of a few hours. If you're already at home, then lucky you! You can crawl straight into bed and get tucked up under the covers and start enjoying your newborn-baby love bubble.

The big day (or night) may be over, but this new chapter is only just beginning . . . and what a brilliant start to it! You will never forget your birth and I hope you never forget what a hero you are, or lose sight of the strength and power you hold within yourself. You brought a human into this world: there's literally nothing you can't do!

12

There's always a plan B . . .

Plan B doesn't have to be second best; plan B can be just as positive, and even better, for you and your baby!

Remember when I said at the beginning of this book that there's always a time and a place for intervention? It would be naive to believe that we will all have the natural, drug-free, intervention-free water birth of our dreams (if, indeed, that even is your dream). Birth can be unpredictable and so too can pregnancy! No amount of relaxation practice will prevent premature rupture of membranes, or pre-eclampsia, gestational diabetes or obstetric cholestasis from developing.

Therefore, with so many variables that we can't control, it's essential to remain open-minded. Of *course*, focus on the birth you want, but know that should things need to change you will be able to navigate those changes with confidence, using your B.R.A.I.N. to make informed decisions, trusting in your own ability to make the best choices for you and your baby. Ultimately, you want to be in a position to bring your baby into this world calmly and with love, feeling relaxed, respected and hugely empowered by the experience, giving yourself and your baby the best start. That is what a positive birth is! And that is what we are all aiming for. I say it time and time again, but the *mechanics* of how a baby enters the world matter little in comparison to how the parent *feels* during their most significant and life-changing moment. It's the feelings (and memories of those feelings) that last a lifetime.

So, when I talk about a birth plan or rather a *set* of birth *preferences* (the latter being my preferred term), it's definitely not about creating one single plan and going into birth wearing blinkers, believing that any deviation from the plan would be negative or, worse, failing in some way. Rather, I want people to go into birth with a document that they have created, in which they outline their preferences for different scenarios.

Back to the power of language! The word 'preferences' carries very different connotations to 'plan'. Stipulating your *preferences* for birth suggests that there is a way that would be your preferred course of action, but that you're open to other ways should they be deemed better or become necessary. A 'plan' on the other hand feels less fluid and more fixed.

Within the birth preferences document, I recommend considering a few different scenarios and outlining your preferences should they occur. For example, if you're planning a home birth you would obviously outline your preferences for how you want that home birth to go, but you might also outline your preferences if you were to transfer into hospital. If you're planning a vaginal birth in a hospital you might also outline your preferences for a gentle caesarean.

I believe it's very beneficial to have considered – and recorded in writing – your preferences for different situations. This is mainly because, in the moment, you might have a wobble; things could be changing quickly, and you don't want the added stress of having to recall things you read in a book sometime before and that sounded like a good idea. You want to be able to present your birth preferences document and feel calm in the knowledge that you've already given your preferences due thought and have recorded how you want things done in this new situation. By doing this, whatever happens, however things pan out on the day, your preferences are going to be met. By actively putting your wishes *in writing,* you're also making it impossible for your wishes to be ignored or sidelined. Whereas, if you're verbally requesting something, it's possible that the message might not be conveyed to the right people, is miscommunicated or completely lost in translation. If you present those providing your care with a clear document outlining your preferences in writing, they have a duty and obligation to follow what you have outlined. They may well want to discuss your preferences and present their opinion or recommendation, but, at the end of the day, they have a duty to respect your wishes. Because it's *your* body, *your* baby, *your* birth and *your* choice. Always.

Ideally, by going through the process of considering other eventualities, even if they are unlikely to happen, you will feel more prepared, informed and confident – ready for anything! Often, it's the unknown that causes us to feel fearful. If you explore your options (knowing that you always have options), make decisions that feel best for you (knowing that they are always yours to make) and outline your preferences to ensure that your wishes are respected, you will hopefully feel less frightened about navigating any changes in your birth. Instead, you'll feel more confident and empowered at the thought of doing so, knowing that you *can* have a positive experience however you bring your baby into the world.

When it comes to writing up your birth preferences I always recommend that you do it *with* your birth partner, so that they feel involved and part of the process (and also so that they're in the best position to advocate for you). If you have the conversations with your birth partner about your choices then they'll have a deeper understanding of your preferences and be in a better position to advocate for you on the day, rather than just reading from a document they have just seen for the first time.

So, after you have finished reading this book, and perhaps conducted your own research too, I would very much recommend taking some time out with your birth partner to create your own birth preferences document together, using all you have learnt, but also tailoring it to your personal situation and circumstances. To help with this, at the back of the book I have included a birth preferences template for you to use and a completed sample copy (my own) for you to use as a reference. I'm not advocating that you follow my preferences, merely including it so you get an idea of what a completed document might look like. Remember, what you are going to write down are *your* preferences for *your* birth; do not be influenced by what others would do or think you should do. Make your own informed decisions.

Once you have completed this task, make sure you print multiple copies. Include a copy with your maternity notes and pack a few more for back-up in your birth bag. As we've discussed, you might have different midwives supporting you throughout your labour, especially if there is a shift change, and you could have doctors involved at various points, so make sure you have enough copies for everyone.

Then, once that's done, you can put all those thoughts about various scenarios to rest and go forth focusing on the birth you want – your 'A plan' as it were.

Knowing that should you need to make some changes during the course of your birth, you have given everything due thought and consideration and knowing it's all there in your birth preferences document *if* needed is reassuring and means there's no need to ponder and linger on these B or C or D plans any more. In fact, once you've done this, don't waste any more time thinking about 'what ifs', but focus very much on the birth you want, working at building those positive associations with birth, just as we have discussed: read positive birth stories, watch positive birth videos, listen to positive affirmations, look at positive birth photography, and so on.

I also think the act of removing thoughts you're holding onto in your mind, which are taking up valuable brain space, and getting them down on paper is a helpful exercise in itself. If you can't sleep at night and you're worrying about remembering something the next day, you might write yourself a little to-do list or add a reminder to your phone. I do this all the time and find it helps me to relax. I think writing out your birth preferences is similarly helpful.

Lastly, I have heard nothing but positive feedback with regard to this birth preferences template. I have even had people tell me that their midwives said it was the most useful birth plan they'd ever seen – comprehensive and clear. I recall being concerned myself when handing my own over that perhaps I would come across as 'bossy', but I was assured quite the opposite – an in-depth set of birth preferences actually helps midwives do their job. After all, midwives are there to support you and are committed to providing you with 'individualised care' – it's their motto! Instead of spending time trying to work out what kind of support you want (and potentially getting it wrong), it's helpful for them to receive a document which clearly and concisely outlines exactly what kind of support you want and how you want things done. They can then follow these guidelines and ensure your preferences are met. They are on your team! So, don't feel nervous about handing over your birth preferences, you can feel assured that they will be well received, and by doing so you will get the support – and birth – you want.

A comprehensive, in-depth set of birth preferences also helps your birth partner to do their job. Having a clear set of preferences makes it easier for the birth partner to advocate for you, because they can see exactly what your wishes are without having to communicate with you and bother you! It also makes it easier for them, because, especially with everything else going on, it's possible to forget things! By having your preferences written out on paper, birth partners can refer to them and ensure nothing important is overlooked.

On the following pages you'll find an example of how I filled in my own birth preferences sheet, and on pages 204–7 I've provided a template for you to fill in your own sheet.

Birth Preferences

Name: Siobhan Miller (she/her)

Contact number: XXXXX XXX XXX

Estimated due date: 01/04/16

Birth place choice: Home

We wish to have a calm, quiet, water birth at home with no intervention. We are using hypnobirthing for our birth and therefore the environment and language are very important to us. Please note that we would appreciate it if you could avoid using the words 'pain' or 'contractions', and instead talk about 'comfort' and 'surges'. I may describe the power and intensity of a surge but I do not wish to think about or feel pain, as I do not believe birth needs to be painful.

MONITORING

Intermittent monitoring with sonicaid

There is no need to ask when you want to listen in. I would prefer not to be asked questions in labour unless necessary.

I wish to be as mobile as possible/ in the pool so only continuously monitored if absolutely necessary. If continuous monitoring is necessary, I would like to use the wireless monitoring if this is available so that I can continue to move about.

IMPORTANT TO KNOW

Medical conditions

Anaphylaxis. I am extremely allergic to certain drugs and carry an epi-pen.

BIRTH PARTNER

We would like to be left alone whenever possible

Name: James Walton (he/him)

Relationship to you: Partner

Contact number: XXXXX XXX XXX

ENVIRONMENT

It is very important to me that the lighting is dimmed throughout

SIGHT/SOUND/SMELL/ TASTE/TOUCH

I would like my own choice of music to be playing (including hypnobirthing audio tracks), battery-operated tea lights on and our essential oils/room spray.

I'd like to use a birth ball and wear my own clothes initially and then use the birth pool when labour is established. I have a TENS machine I can use in early labour and plan to eat and drink normally.

PAIN RELIEF

Please do not offer any to me

I do not wish to have an epidural. I do not want Pethidine/Diamorphine or any other drugs. I do not like gas and air because it makes me sick. Ideally I do not want any drugs introduced during my labour or afterwards.

Please remind me of the tools I do have which include: my breathing techniques, visualisations (of a balloon filling as I inhale and a golden thread as I exhale), light-touch massage, heat pack, cold flannel, essential oils, relaxation scripts, relaxation audio tracks, positive affirmations, the pool, etc. These will all increase my comfort level.

Please remind me of my desire to feel and experience this birth and of my previous positive birth experience if I have a wobble.

POSITIONS FOR LABOUR & BIRTH

I do not wish to be lying on my back

I would like to be active and use positions that mean I am upright, forward and open (U.F.O.) which facilitate an easier and quicker birth. I'd like to remain mobile throughout. If I need to rest, I would like to use my birthing ball or lean over the sofa/bed. In the pool I wish to be upright and leaning forward over the side or on all fours.

BIRTH POOL

I would like to use the birthing pool during labour and would like to give birth in the pool.

SECOND STAGE

I do not want to be coached to push

I would like to breathe my baby down so they are born gently and calmly. I would like to follow the lead of my body rather than be coached to push.

I would like to be able to bring my baby to my chest immediately after delivery. If it is not possible for me to hold the baby then I would like the baby to have skin-to-skin time with my birth partner.

It is important that the calm and intimate environment is maintained after baby has been born as this helps with the flow of oxytocin which aids bonding and reduces the risk of excessive blood loss and PND.

LABOUR WARD

Private room, birth pool, low lighting, hushed voices

If I birth my baby in hospital I would like to request a private room with a birthing pool. The environment is very important to us so we would like the room to be as similar as possible to our preferences outlined for home birth.

Most importantly we would like the room to be dimly lit, quiet and with as few people as possible present.

We would like people to knock before entering and to speak in hushed voices. All communication is to go through my birth partner please so that I can labour undisturbed.

I do not wish for students to be present, only hospital staff who absolutely need to be there.

I do not wish to be cannulated unless it is essential to do so.

ASSISTED DELIVERY

I will accept assistance if there is no other option

I would rather wait longer than try to rush the process unless the baby is in obvious distress and needs to be born.

THIRD STAGE

'The Golden Hour' – baby on my chest immediately after birth and undisturbed skin-to-skin time for an hour

It is my preference to have a physiological third stage. I would like to wait until my baby has received all of their blood before the cord is clamped and cut. I would like to birth the placenta without any drugs being introduced to my body.

I am having my placenta encapsulated so please be mindful of this. It will need to be stored in a sterile container which we will provide and placed in the fridge/cool box within half an hour.

In the event that I experience a postpartum haemorrhage, I accept that I will need to have the injection. If I continue to lose blood then I accept I will need to transfer to a labour ward to receive syntocinon via a drip.

UNPLANNED CAESAREAN

Gentle/natural cesarean please!

If I choose to birth my baby by caesarean, it would be my preference to have a gentle or natural caesarean and to be awake for this.

I would like to receive my baby to my chest immediately after delivery, certainly before they are weighed or cleaned.

Please ensure any electrodes are placed on my back so they are not in the way and do not inhibit this important skin-to-skin time.

I would like my baby to receive all of their blood so wish to request delayed cord clamping.

I wish for only those who are absolutely necessary to be present in theatre.

I would like to be able to see my baby be born so please lower the curtain at this stage.

I would appreciate it if the lights could be dimmed at head end so when the baby is delivered and brought to my chest, they are not subjected to bright light.

I would like my choice of music/ relaxation track to be playing in theatre during the birth of my baby.

If there is time beforehand, I would like to be given a pack of sterile gauze strips so that I have the opportunity to seed my baby with bacteria and stimulate microbiome development, which would happen if they were born vaginally.

I would still like my placenta to be encapsulated after birth, so please bear this in mind and ensure the theatre staff are aware of my wishes. My placenta will need to be stored in a sterile container and kept cool until collected.

If my baby has to be in the Special Care Unit, then I want to be able to care for them as much as possible and to ensure they receive my breast milk. I would like help with making sure this happens.

ANYTHING ELSE . . .

I am happy for my baby to be given Vitamin K by injection.

I plan to breastfeed and **feel confident doing so**.

If I am admitted to the postnatal ward I would like a private room if one is available.

THANK YOU

Thank you for taking the time to read my birth preferences. I am looking forward to the birth of my baby and planning for a positive and empowering birth experience where my baby is born safely and calmly. I believe this is possible however my birth story pans out.

Thank you for supporting us at this very special time in our lives. We will be sure to appreciate all you do for us, now and for the rest of time.

Siobhan and James

Birth Preferences

Name:

Contact number:

Estimated due date:

Birth place choice:

IMPORTANT TO KNOW

BIRTH PARTNER

Name:

Relationship to you:

Contact number:

ENVIRONMENT

MONITORING

PAIN RELIEF

SECOND STAGE

LABOUR WARD

POSITIONS FOR LABOUR & BIRTH

BIRTH POOL

ASSISTED DELIVERY

UNPLANNED CAESAREAN

THIRD STAGE

ANYTHING ELSE . . .

THANK YOU

BIRTH STORY

Planned, unscheduled caesarean – Verity, first-time parent

We discovered our baby was breech at thirty-seven weeks, which somewhat changed our vision of a beautiful, calm hypnobirth in water. Despite two ECVs, reflexology, acupuncture, the Webster technique, days spent doing inversions and, of course, lots of hypnobirthing visualisations, it became clear that they had chosen their position and weren't budging. Whilst a vaginal breech birth was an option, we didn't feel that the expertise was guaranteed at our hospital and, being so late in the day, there wasn't the time to find an alternative. We decided that an elective caesarean was the safest way to bring our baby into the world. However, we also decided, after much research, that we wanted our baby to choose their birthday – opting for a planned but unscheduled, natural caesarean. We discovered that there are numerous benefits of labouring a little, both for parent and baby (in low-risk situations), rather than going with the medical status quo of scheduled C-section at thirty-nine weeks. Needless to say, this made us deeply unpopular with our hospital and the last few weeks were a bit of an emotional rollercoaster, with a lot of pressure on us to book in for the caesarean. We eventually set ourselves a cut off of forty-one weeks, where we felt that the risks of waiting would start outweighing the benefits of spontaneous labour. Our baby arrived at forty weeks and six days.

The caesarean itself was beautiful – all the scaremongering about it becoming an emergency couldn't have been further from the reality. I woke up with surges at 7am and we calmly went into the hospital at 9am, went into theatre at 12.30pm, and our baby was born at 1.15pm. Very aptly, Take That's 'Patience' was playing on the radio at the time . . . We got the slow, gentle caesarean we had planned for with delayed cord clamping, immediate skin-to-skin and a quiet, peaceful theatre. It might not have been option A, but we are so grateful for all the support we had in adapting our preferences and still making it a beautiful experience and peaceful way to welcome our baby into the world. The course, all the hypnobirthing practice and Siobhan's guidance and encouragement made a huge difference.

13

Packing the ultimate birth bag

If this is your first birth experience, chances are you have already spent some time thinking about your 'birth bag' – or 'hospital bag' as it's more commonly referred to. You might have done some research and read some of the endless lists available online and wondered how everything was supposed to fit in one single bag (spoiler: it doesn't!). If this is your second, third, fourth or even fifth birth, it could be that packing the birth bag is a bit of a last-minute afterthought. Either way, I do believe that the physical packing of the bag and the mental preparation involved in doing so is an important process to go through in advance of birth.

I call it a birth bag because of course not everyone is going to hospital, and, even if you are, it's a bag full of items for you to use in *birth*, not items specific for a hospital! Also, more significantly, considering the power of language, referring to the birth bag as a 'hospital bag' conjures up images of hospital stays and illness. A hospital bag is normally packed if you are going to stay in hospital after a medical procedure and so carries these associations. If you're planning for a positive and magical birth experience you'd benefit from having a different mindset.

I also recommend packing a birth bag, even if you don't plan on going anywhere! If you're planning a home birth, I believe it's 100 per cent still worth packing a bag. There are a few reasons for this.

1. You could end up transferring into the hospital for some reason, either in labour or afterwards. The risk of transfer because of an emergency is very low, but the transfer rate for first-time parents from home or birth centres into hospital is actually quite high – around 50 per cent. The most common reasons for transfer are requiring stronger pain relief (epidural), slow progress and meconium in the waters. Given that this *could* happen, it's worth having the bag packed and ready to go.

2. If you birth at home and remain at home, you're still going to want to have everything you need to hand. Packing everything into a birth bag means your birth partner can easily locate the items you need, rather than having to leave your side every so often to go and hunt around the house for them. Having everything in one place, in one bag, is helpful for everyone.

3. I believe the act of packing the bag offers some psychological benefits. You're taking time out of your day to do a mindful activity that is about preparing for birth and meeting your baby. You are taking the opportunity to think carefully about how things are going to pan out (positive visualisation) and packing the items you think you'll need at the various points. By doing this you will start to feel more prepared, ready and excited for what lies ahead.

When you come to pack the bag, I like to think of it as packing for a spa break or luxury weekend away! This might seem bizarre, and you're probably wondering how those huge absorbent maternity pads that you need to pack fit with the image of a regular spa break, but bear with me ... breast pads and maternity pads aside, you should be packing items that will make you feel good and help you to relax. Little treats, for example! Your comfiest clothes! You should feel excited when labour begins, excited to meet your baby, but also a little bit excited to crack open your bag of goodies and dig in! Giving birth is such a special, magical time – treat it as such when packing your bag. You are going to be doing something monumental, so if there was ever the time for a little self-indulgence, it is now.

Also, remember the environment and the five senses checklist. So, your room spray or essential oils (smell), music, headphones, portable speaker (sound), battery-operated tea lights or fairy lights, an eye mask (sight), decent tea bags (NHS ones are not the best if you're a fan of a strong cuppa), snacks (taste), massage oil, fluffy socks, slippers, bikini, cosy dressing gown, oversized comfy tee, your own pillow, blanket (touch). Never underestimate the environment, set the scene for the birth you want!

You'll notice in the packing list opposite, I've put all of the stuff you might need to transform the environment under the birth partner's checklist – this is because it's your birth partner who will likely be setting up the room when you're in established labour. Hence, it makes sense for them to have all the bits to do this in *their* bag, so they can take charge and easily lay their hands on everything they need.

So without further ado here's my packing list for 'the *ultimate* birth bag':

BIRTHING PARENT	BIRTH PARTNER
❑ Pregnancy notes	❑ Hypnobirthing book
❑ Copies of Birth Preferences	❑ Relaxation MP3s and music
❑ Large T-shirt to wear in labour	❑ Wireless speaker and charger
❑ Eye mask	❑ iPhone and charger
❑ iPhone, charger and headphones	❑ Camera and charger
❑ Swimwear if desired for a birth pool	❑ Battery-operated tea lights
❑ Slippers	❑ Fairy lights
❑ Dressing gown	❑ Room fragrance/pillow spray
❑ Fluffy socks	❑ Massage oil
❑ Snacks (non-perishable)	❑ Essential oils, e.g. lavender
❑ Drinks (coconut water is great)	❑ Swimwear if going in a birth pool
❑ Flannels	❑ Snacks and drinks for yourself
❑ Facial spray/spritzer	❑ Toothbrush, toothpaste, deodorant
❑ Lip balm	❑ Change for parking (if needed)
❑ Water bottle with straw	❑ Mini bottle of champagne!
❑ Thick headband and hair bands	
❑ Your pillow	**BABY**
❑ TENS machine (if using)	
❑ Hot water bottle or wheat bag	❑ Nappies (allow ten a day)
❑ Positive affirmation cards	❑ Cotton wool balls (use with water – avoid using wipes at first)
❑ Birth ball (if needed)	❑ Olive oil in small bottle (apply to baby's bum before nappy – it will make cleaning much easier!)
❑ Two nursing bras	
❑ Breast pads	
❑ Nipple cream (lansinoh is good)	
❑ Maternity pads (two packs)	❑ Three cotton sleepsuits with feet
❑ Plenty of big cotton pants	
❑ Front-opening nightie or PJs	❑ Three cotton vests
❑ Toiletries and make-up	❑ Two hats
❑ Towel	❑ Muslin squares
❑ Hairbrush	❑ Baby blanket
❑ Comfy outfit for going home	❑ Jacket or snowsuit if winter
	❑ Infant car seat

14

Conclusion
You've got this!

And so, you have reached the end! Not the 'end' end of course – just the end of this book. You're actually now at the beginning of the most immense new chapter of your life. Having read this book, you have already begun preparing for your amazing birth experience. You are now on the cusp (or at least approaching it) of experiencing something really incredible and life-changing! Honestly, I get goosebumps just writing and thinking about this. Giving birth – however you choose to do it – is truly the most amazing thing you will ever experience in your life, and meeting your precious baby for the first time is one of life's most unforgettable moments. And then, from that point onwards, whether it's your first baby or your fourth, your life changes for-ever as you embark on the journey of raising this small person. A journey that no doubt will test you at points, but one that will also give you the highest of highs as you experience more love and joy than you ever thought possible. Your heart will expand. And right now, you are on your way to experiencing all of this. I am so excited for you ... in fact, I'll admit, part of me wishes I was you!

At the beginning of this book you might remember I mentioned the 'anxiety to excitement' spectrum that I believe everyone sits on. At the start some people might have felt very anxious about birth – terrified, even – whereas others might already have been feeling pretty excited. I said I hoped, no matter where you were on the spectrum initially, that you would have moved towards 'excitement' by the time you reached the end of this book. Now that we've arrived at this point I truly hope you are aware of a shift within yourself and are feeling – or at least beginning to feel – excited for your birth and, dare I say it, looking forward to the experience. Perhaps you can take a moment to reflect on where you started and where you are now . . .

I hope you now feel better informed about all aspects of birth, more confident in your amazing body, empowered by the knowledge that you have ownership over all decisions relating to your body and your birth and, finally, well prepared with a whole host of practical tools you can use to navigate whatever lies ahead. Best of all, I hope you are excited to meet your baby and start your journey in the best way possible: calmly, confidently, happily and full of love.

Before I sign off, just as I do when teaching classes, I urge you to take what you have learnt and act on it right away. No delay and no excuses! Life is busy, and I know first-hand how easy it is to defer getting started on something because you feel you're at full capacity already. But this is important and really will make your birth better. I don't say that lightly. The practice or the 'homework', if you will, takes just fifteen minutes a day and is well worth it. You have already invested a great deal of your time in reading this book, so now is the time to ensure your input has been worth it. Ideally the reading alone has initiated a shift in your mindset, but please do go on and build upon this as your pregnancy progresses; the more practice you do, the more you reinforce what you have learnt, the more effective everything will be and the better you will feel today, tomorrow, when you give birth and for all the years that follow.

Please don't worry if you're reading this and don't have long to go – everything you have learnt in this book will help you, and the hypnobirthing tools and relaxation techniques will make a big difference at whatever point you begin using them. Best of all, if you do give birth shortly, everything is likely to be very fresh in your mind!

So now you're on board and keen to get started, here's what you could do right now, today ...

Read a positive birth story
Watch a positive birth video
Look at positive birth photography
Listen to positive affirmations
Make or buy some positive affirmation cards

Links to all of the above can be found in the resources section at the back of this book, making it really very easy to get started.

Next, look at the practice schedule I have created (also included at the back of this book) and aim to begin tonight: just a few repetitions of the up breathing followed by a guided relaxation exercise or light-touch massage before bed. You could then drift off to sleep listening to some relaxation MP3s or music. The more you do this, the more familiar it will all become and the easier it will be for you to access that 'green state' of deep relaxation in labour – and life! You will most likely really enjoy the practice and find it offers you immediate benefits (more relaxed, less anxious, better sleep and so on), which will encourage you to keep going. And once you get started, I hope it will become part of your normal evening routine, as regular as brushing your teeth.

Finally, go out there (in person or online) and engage with

people and communities who share and celebrate positive birth stories. The more you immerse yourself in this positive environment, the more confident you will become and the more supported you will feel as you move closer to giving birth. You'll also start to realise that, contrary to the tales you might have been told (or the stories you've been sold by the media), people are in fact having amazing births every single day!

You'll find that if you speak to people who have had positive birth experiences, they'll likely tell you that they'd jump at the chance to get to do it again! I certainly feel that way. And as one person said in their birth story, 'a positive birth leaves you on a high you feel you might never come down from'. Giving birth is truly life-altering and life-expanding; you tap into a power and strength you may not have even realised you had. And once you realise you are in fact a legitimate superhero, you never forget it. You carry the strength with you always; so whenever times are tough, you can remind yourself how strong and capable you really are. Nobody can ever take a positive and empowering birth experience away from you. That is something you carry with you for life.

Finally, I am going to say goodbye and thank you. Thank you for buying this book, thank you for being brave enough to challenge the cultural status quo and believe that birth can be better – because it really can. Not just better, but amazing! Thank you for the time you've spent on my words. I have put everything I know about birth into this book, learned through years of studying, teaching and my own experiences, and have tried to make it as accessible as possible. Hypnobirthing has been life-changing for me and I hope with all my heart that this book has been useful to read. And maybe even life-changing for you too.

Siobhan x

Guided relaxation scripts

Below you will find three scripts for you to use with your birth partner as part of your daily relaxation practice. Aim to do one script a day, ideally before bed, or alternatively ten minutes of light-touch massage. Remember, you'll find a practice schedule to help you out at the back of the book.

These scripts can be referred to as guided meditations, but you can also call them guided relaxation exercises if you prefer. You don't need to be experienced with meditation – or even into meditation – to find these scripts helpful. All you need to do is set aside some time with your birth partner (approximately fifteen minutes is all you need) so that they can read the script to you whilst you close your eyes and focus on the words that are being spoken. It's ok if your mind drifts and you begin to think of something else, so long as you recognise this has happened and return your focus to the script. The more you practise, the quicker you will find you can zone everything out and access that 'green' state of deep relaxation that feels so good. Doing this is essentially mindfulness practice – when you take time out to slow everything down, reduce the noisy chatter in your mind, and focus on the present – and is known to offer numerous mental health benefits. You may well continue this practice long after your baby is born, if it's not something you do already. But even if you don't, you should notice immediate benefits when you practise now in pregnancy. It's not something you have to do in the hope it pays off; it should help right away by giving you a way to relax, helping you feel more connected to your birth partner and helping you to sleep better.

The first 'simple guided relaxation' is the most straight-forward and a good place to start. Your birth partner simply needs to read the script (the text in *italics*) as it's written on the page. It's best if they read it slowly (the slower the better!) in a calm, hushed voice. It doesn't matter if they aren't used to reading such things and, sure, you may have a giggle when you first begin! But you will both soon get the hang of it. You can reassure your birth partner by letting them know that they are better than any recorded MP3 you could get because their voice is *familiar*. And it's that familiarity which will bring you comfort and help you to relax.

Simple guided relaxation

Allow your eyes to close gently and easily, so that you are better able to focus on my voice. Feel your body begin to relax.

Tune in now with your breath. Allow it to slow down and deepen. Settle into a rhythm that feels natural for you. Breathe slowly, deeply and comfortably.

As you inhale, feel your lungs gently expand and, as you exhale, imagine that a valve has opened, and you feel all the pressure within you release. Now, again. Inhale, expand, exhale, release. Feel all the tension flow out and away from your body. Breathe in and breathe out. Inhale, expand. Exhale, release. Allow everything to soften, relax and release ... You feel completely comfortable ... You are totally relaxed ...

Focus now on your eyelids and allow the muscles to soften. Feel the relaxation spreads upwards and across your forehead. Everything softening and relaxing. Feel the muscles relax so that your forehead is smooth and free of all tension. Allow yourself to sink into this lovely feeling of warmth and comfort as everything becomes soft and relaxed. Inhale, expand. Exhale, release. Breathe in and breathe out. Enjoy this feeling of peace, calm and well-being.

Now feel the relaxation spread downwards from your forehead, in and around your eyes and down through your cheeks. Everything softens as the warm feeling gently spreads. Allow your jaw to become loose so that it too is relaxed. Feel the warmth spread on downwards through your neck and across your shoulders. All the muscles soften and release as the relaxation gently spreads downwards through your body. Everything is loose and relaxed.

Notice now your mouth and your lips. Allow them to soften and release. Notice your tongue – it rests completely relaxed in your mouth. Every muscle in your face is soft and free of tension. Your whole face and head feel completely relaxed. Inhale, expand. Exhale, release. Breathe in and breathe out. You feel very, very peaceful.

Finally, feel your shoulders relax. Allow them to sink to their natural level, so that your whole body is limp and relaxed, and your breathing is soft and slow. Pause for a moment and enjoy this feeling of calm, warmth and well-being.

You feel happy now, knowing that you can easily access this wonderful feeling of peace, calm and relaxation whenever you need to. You know that your body has been perfectly designed to grow and birth your baby. You feel strong and confident, calm and relaxed. You know that you can feel just as relaxed as you do now when you give birth to your baby, and so you look forward to meeting your baby feeling calm and full of love. You look forward to the amazing and empowering experience that is giving birth, trusting that you, your body and your baby know exactly what to do.

Now, when you're ready, and in your own time, slowly open your eyes, gently and calmly, coming back to the present feeling relaxed, confident and ready.

✻

The next script, 'arm-stroking guided relaxation', also involves reading the script slowly and calmly, but also includes an additional element: arm stroking. Your birth partner simply needs to stroke your hand and arm whilst reading the script, when directed to do so. How lightly or firmly they stroke should be dictated by your personal preference, but they should aim to stroke the arm back and forth nice and slowly.

Arm-stroking guided relaxation

Gently and easily allow your eyes to close so that you can focus on my voice and begin to relax.

Allow your breathing to slow down and deepen. As you inhale, feel your lungs expand as they fill with air, and as you exhale, feel all the pressure and tension release and flow out of your body. Inhale, expand. Exhale, release. Breathing in and breathing out. With each breath you become more and more relaxed. Inhale, expand. Exhale, release. Breathing in and breathing out. You feel peaceful. You feel comfortable. You feel deeply relaxed.

Now place your focus on your feet. Feel the weight of your feet where they rest. As you focus on your feet, imagine all the stress and tension in your body draining out through them, down, down and away, into the ground. You begin to feel lighter. Everything feels more relaxed.

Now imagine that as all the stress and tension leave your body, a wave of relaxation and peace flows down through you. You can feel this wave of warmth and light as it slowly spreads and fills every part of your body. You feel an overwhelming feeling of comfort and well-being as this wave of peace and relaxation, warmth and light, fills every part of you.

You breathe slowly and deeply. Inhale, expand. Exhale, release. Breathing in and breathing out. Slower and deeper.

Now that you are relaxed, I will begin to stroke your hand and arm very gently.

[Start stroking their hand and arm, speaking slowly and calmly.]

You can feel my touch on your hand and arm. I am here. You are safe. Allow yourself to sink, deeply relaxed, completely comfortable. As I stroke your hand and arm you relax more and more deeply. You can feel my touch. It feels soothing and reassuring. You are completely safe.

Enjoy this feeling. Endorphins spreading throughout your body. Inhale, expand. Exhale, release. Breathing in and breathing out. You are deeply relaxed. Peaceful and calm. Filled with warmth and light.

Now the feeling in your hand and arm begins to fade. You know that I am still stroking your hand and arm ... but all you can feel is warmth and comfort. Maybe you can feel a light tingle from my touch, but as I continue to stroke, the feeling becomes less and less. Your hand and arm become increasingly numb.

Inhale, expand. Exhale, release. Inhale. Exhale. Breathing in and breathing out.

You feel more and more deeply relaxed. You are completely comfortable. Peaceful. Safe. Gradually the feeling in your hand and arm becomes less and less. Fading away. Until you feel nothing at all.

Inhale, expand. Exhale, release. Breathing in and breathing out.

You realise now that you can move this warm, comfortable feeling of numbness wherever you want. Simply focus on a part of your body and the feeling becomes less and less, gradually fades away ... until there is nothing at all.

Enjoy this sensation that fills your body ... Warmth and light. Peace and calm.

You are now very, very relaxed.

Just pause and enjoy this wonderful feeling of well-being, peace and calm that fills your body.

You know now that you are a strong, powerful and capable person and are perfectly designed to grow and birth your baby.

You appreciate the power of your intuition, and you trust that it will guide you through your labour and birth.

You know that birth is safe and you are safe.

You understand how important it is to be relaxed when giving birth and you feel confident that you are able to access this deep relaxation when needed.

You understand your mind and body are connected so you prepare mentally for the positive and empowering birth experience you wish for.

You know that the decisions in birth are yours to make and you feel empowered by this fact.

You look forward to meeting your baby and holding them in your arms.

[Stop stroking.]

Inhale, expand. Exhale, release. Breathing in and breathing out.

This relaxation has been very powerful. You feel relaxed, calm and peaceful. You now know that you have power to control the sensations in your body.

In a moment it will be time to come back to the present, slowly and gently. You feel calm, relaxed and confident. And each time you do this, these feelings will grow stronger and stronger. You will become more and more confident and you will be able to access this deep relaxation more quickly than before.

So now, in your own time, come back to the present, slowly and gently opening your eyes, feeling calm, relaxed and confident.

*

The final script, the 'arm-drop and release guided relaxation', is again to be read slowly and calmly. It includes an arm-drop element which helps you to let go of any tension you're holding onto and to deepen your relaxation throughout your body. Your birth partner simply needs to lift your arm gently at the wrist and let it fall into your lap when directed to do so.

These last two scripts require some multitasking skills, but hopefully nothing beyond anyone's capabilities. However, to make things easier, you could get your birth partner to record their voice reading the script (on their phone, perhaps) and then play this whilst they focus on the arm stroking or the arm drop. You could then also listen to the recording if your birth partner is not with you when you come to do your practice, but still benefit from hearing their familiar voice.

Arm-drop and release guided relaxation

[Gently rest your hand on their bump]

As my hand rests here, allow your eyes to close, gently and easily, so that you can better focus on my voice. Feel the muscles in your eyelids soften and relax, so that your eyelids feel light and your forehead is soft and smooth.

Tune in now with your breathing. Allow your breath to slow down and deepen. Inhale, feel your lungs expand. Exhale, feel all tension release. Breathing in and breathing out. Feel all your tension and stress flow out of your body and away.

Focus now on your eyes – they feel relaxed. Feel your cheeks soften, allow your lips to part and your jaw to rest, loose and relaxed.

Now allow your shoulders to sink to their natural level as you feel the relaxation spread down your neck, across your shoulders and on down through your back. You feel calm, relaxed and peaceful.

Your whole body sinks into the lovely, familiar feeling of warm relaxation. You are completely comfortable. You know that you are safe.

You relax deeper and deeper. It feels so good to take the time to just allow everything to soften, release and relax. So comfortable, so easy. Embrace this wonderful feeling of warmth and well-being.

Inhale, expand. Exhale, release. Breathing in and breathing out.

You feel the relaxation slowly spreading throughout your body until every single cell feels soft and relaxed. You feel so calm and peaceful, happy and relaxed.

And every time you feel my hand rest here, you will recognise this as a sign to let go and relax. You know you can access this wonderful feeling any time you wish.

Tune in again with your breathing. Breathe slowly and deeply. Inhale, expand. Exhale, release. Breathing in and breathing out. So comfortable, so relaxed.

Now I shall lift your arm gently at the wrist. Just relax and let me take all of the weight. [Raise arm]

Notice how heavy your arm feels. It feels so good to just relax and allow me to take the weight.

In a moment, I will gently release your arm and it will fall, landing in your lap, and your relaxation will deepen even more. [Let go of arm]

Now, again, I will lift your arm, slowly and gently. Feel the weight of your arm as I raise it. [Raise arm] *You are completely relaxed.*

In a moment I will let your arm go again and, as I do, your relaxation will become even deeper and more profound. [Let go of arm] *You are now so deeply relaxed.*

And again, one last time, I'm lifting your arm. [Raise arm] *You allow me to take the full weight of your arm. As I let go, your arm falls into your lap and you go many times deeper.* [Let go of arm]

Rest now, comfortable and relaxed. Enjoy the feeling of calm and well-being that radiates throughout your body.

Know that this easy, deep relaxation is there for you when it comes to labour and birth. Know that you can feel just as calm and relaxed then as you do right now.

You know that your body has been perfectly designed to grow and birth your baby, easily and comfortably. You look forward to giving birth to your baby because you know it is going to be the most amazing and empowering experience, and you will meet your baby feeling calm and confident, happy and relaxed.

Now the time has come to return to the present, slowly and gently, allow your eyes to open and return, feeling confident and relaxed about birth, bringing with you all the lovely feelings of calm and contentment you have just created.

*

Hypnobirthing Practice Schedule

	Monday	Tuesday	Wednesday	Thursday	Friday	Saturday	Sunday
daytime	positive statements, birth stories & videos	positive statements, birth stories & videos	positive statements, birth stories & videos	positive statements, birth stories & videos	positive statements, birth stories & videos	positive statements, birth stories & videos	positive statements, birth stories & videos
daytime	practise down breathing on toilet	practise down breathing on toilet	practise down breathing on toilet	practise down breathing on toilet	practise down breathing on toilet	practise down breathing on toilet	practise down breathing on toilet
evening	practise up breathing before relaxation exercise	practise up breathing before relaxation exercise	practise up breathing before relaxation exercise	practise up breathing before relaxation exercise	practise up breathing before relaxation exercise	practise up breathing before relaxation exercise	practise up breathing before relaxation exercise
evening	simple guided relaxation	10 mins of light-touch massage	arm-stroking guided relaxation	arm-drop and release guided relaxation	10 mins of light-touch massage	simple guided relaxation	10 mins of light-touch massage
bedtime	play relaxation mp3s	play relaxation mp3s	play relaxation mp3s	play relaxation mp3s	play relaxation mp3s	play relaxation mp3s	play relaxation mp3s

Resources

UP BREATHING AND DOWN BREATHING

If you want to see up and down breathing in action, I've made some demonstration videos to help you with your practice. You'll find them, along with a few others, on my YouTube channel: www.youtube.com/thepositivebirthcompany

GUIDED MEDITATIONS AND POSITIVE AFFIRMATIONS

You'll find a selection of MP3s that I've recorded, plus my Little Pack of Positivity (positive affirmation cards to place around your home) available to download and buy here: www.thepositivebirthcompany.co.uk/shop. For more general guided relaxation (not specifically for pregnancy) Headspace is a very popular app.

SURGE TIMER

I've created a hypnobirthing-friendly virtual birth partner app to support you through birth and help you keep track of your surges. It's called 'Freya' and can be downloaded from both the App Store and Google Play Store. The app will coach you through your surges by counting for you, and – when in surge mode – you will see an expanding circle visualisation, which you can also breathe in sync with. Between surges you can listen to guided relaxations, positive affirmations, music of your choice and voice notes from friends and family. You can visit the log at any point to see how frequently your surges are coming and how long they are lasting.

POSITIVE BIRTH STORIES

You'll find lots of real-life, positive, inspiring and reassuring birth stories on my blog here: www.thepositivebirthcompany.co.uk/ blog and you'll also find lots more on Instagram by searching the campaign hashtag #PositiveBirthStoryProject. Please do join in with the campaign by sharing and celebrating your own story when the time comes using #PositiveBirthStoryProject and help show the world that birth can be a wonderful experience.

HYPNOBIRTHING DIGITAL PACK

The Hypnobirthing Digital Pack is the world's most affordable, accessible and inclusive online hypnobirthing programme, created as part of my mission to make hypnobirthing more accessible for all. The Hypnobirthing Digital Pack offers you the full course in video format and is available to watch on demand on any device from anywhere in the world at any time of day or night. It includes MP3s to download, plus a course notes booklet, an infant feeding guide and an editable birth preferences template as well as access to a private online community for ongoing support www.thepositivebirthcompany. co.uk/digital-pack

POSITIVE BIRTH VIDEOS AND PHOTOGRAPHY

YouTube is a great resource for positive birth videos. If you visit The Positive Birth Company channel you will find a playlist of my favourite birth videos: www.youtube.com/thepositive-birthcompany. Once you start watching, YouTube will begin recommending other similar videos for you to see. Instagram is a great resource for positive birth photography. You'll find lots of wonderful images on The Positive Birth Company page: www.instagram.com/thepositivebirthcompany

OTHER RESOURCES

NICE guidelines: www.nice.org.uk
Evidence-based Birth: evidencebasedbirth.com
Choosing your birth place: https://www.birthrights.org.uk/factsheets/choice-of-place-of-birth/
Having a baby if you're LGBT+: https://www.nhs.uk/pregnancy/having-a-baby-if-you-are-lgbt-plus/
Doulas: https://doula.org.uk/about-doulas

References

The Science Stuff

1 www.babycenter.com/0_preterm-labor-test-fetal-fibronectin_1511.bc
2 Dick-Read, G. (2004) *Childbirth without fear: the principles and practice of natural childbirth.* Pinter & Martin: London.

The Toolkit

3 Hill, Milli (2017) *The Positive Birth Book: A New Approach to Pregnancy, Birth and the Early Weeks.* Pinter & Martin Ltd.

Choosing where to give birth

4 www.which.co.uk/birth-choice/units/london
5 www.npeu.ox.ac.uk/birthplace
6 www.npeu.ox.ac.uk/birthplace
7 www.npeu.ox.ac.uk/birthplace
8 www.npeu.ox.ac.uk/birthplace
9 www.which.co.uk/birth-choice
10 www.nice.org.uk/guidance/cg190/chapter/recommendations

Bring it on baby! Induction

11 www.nice.org.uk/guidance/cg70/chapter/Introduction
12 www.nice.org.uk/guidance/cg70/chapter/Introduction
13 evidencebasedbirth.com/evidence-on-inducing-labor-for-going-past-your-due-date

14 evidencebasedbirth.com/evidence-on-inducing-labor-for-going-past-your-due-date

15 evidencebasedbirth.com/evidence-on-inducing-labor-for-going-past-your-due-date

16 www.nice.org.uk/guidance/cg70/chapter/1-guidance

17 www.nice.org.uk/advice/esnm38/chapter/introduction

Go Gentle: Opting for a natural caesarean

18 www.bmj.com/content/343/bmj.d7400

Index

(page numbers in *italic* represent diagrams; those in **bold** represent tables and lists)

Acknowledgements

I really cannot believe I have written an actual book. I was an avid reader as a child – a real bookworm who rebelled by staying up past lights-out with a book, tilting it towards the crack in my bedroom door so the light from the hallway would offer enough illumination to enable me to continue reading. My love of books extended well into my teenage years and led me to study English Literature for my first degree. To have been given the opportunity to write a book and be published has been a dream come true; a huge tick on the dream-life bucket list.

A large number of people have made this possible and the hardest bit about writing these acknowledgements is the real fear that I will forget to thank someone integral! So, pre-empting this, I would like first to offer a massive and general (albeit very sincere!) thank-you to every single person who has, in whatever way, helped this book come to be a real-life published piece of work. That said, there are a few people who deserve an extra special thank-you and to be named individually for their efforts . . .

Zoe, Emily, Jillian, Jo and the rest of the team at Little, Brown, thank you for your patience and encouragement and for being as passionate and excited about this book as I am. Thanks to Louise Turpin and Josephine Dellow for the interior illustrations, and Hannah Wood for the cover design. Thanks to my agent Hannah Ferguson, and my friend (and author) Sarah Turner for introducing us. You both have kept me going when the overwhelm has peaked. Thank you. To my friend Lucy Flower for recommending me to her friend Alyson Slater who, in turn, recommended me to her cousin Lucy Malagoni, who then said, 'I've a colleague who might be interested in your book idea.' Without that happy chain of events this book would likely not exist.

Thank you to Oisin, Arlo and Ailbe Fox, to whom this book is dedicated, for making me a mum – this book, my business, none of it exists without you. I *promise* to spend more time being Mum and less time writing and working from now on. To James, my partner in birth, parenting and life, thank you for stepping up when I started working on my business and stepping up again when I also took on writing a book; for running the home and raising the children almost single-handedly, making me endless cups of tea and margaritas, allowing me to lie in after I'd spent all night awake (a frequent occurrence) and reminding me that I could do this, whenever I doubted myself (which was often). All this whilst holding down your own full-time job. Thank you for enabling me and encouraging me to do this (and hardly ever berating me for taking on too much)! And to my brother Mike, who insists I mention him, for championing me always and letting me know how proud he is of his big sis.

Finally, my biggest thank-you goes to the thousands of amazing and inspiring people I have had the honour of teaching – some of whom have contributed their birth stories for inclusion in this book. I am so grateful to each and every one of you for allowing me to play a small part in the most magical chapter of your lives. I am truly privileged and forever grateful for your support, which has been immense and genuinely life-changing for me.